PSYCHOANALYSIS AND FILM

PSYCHOANALYSIS AND FILM

Edited and with an Introduction by Glen O. Gabbard

International Journal of Psychoanalysis Key Papers Series
Series Editor: Paul Williams

London and New York
KARNAC

First published in 2001 by
H. Karnac (Books) Ltd
6 Pembroke Buildings, London NW 10 6RE
A subsidiary of Other Press LLC, New York.

British Library Cataloguing in Publication Data.

A C.I.P. for this book is available from the British Library.

ISBN 1 85575 275 1

Edited and typeset by the *International Journal of Psychoanalysis*

www.karnacbooks.com

CONTENTS:

1. INTRODUCTION

GLEN O. GABBARD

In 1895 there were two auspicious births. The Lumière brothers invented a rudimentary film projector, signifying the birth of the cinema, and *Studies in Hysteria* appeared, inaugurating the new science of psychoanalysis. Throughout the twentieth century the two new disciplines have been inextricably linked. As early as 1900 a writer would describe his psychotic episode in terms of 'the magic lantern' effects of the nickelodeons (Schneider, 1985). By 1916 Harvard psychologist Hugo Münsterberg was applying psychological understanding to the study of the cinema. He suggested that 'the photo play' more or less replicated the mechanisms of the mind in a way that was more compelling than the typical narrative forms of storytelling. In 1931 the American film industry was already being called a 'dream factory' (Ehrenburg, 1931), reflecting the close resemblance between film imagery and the work of dreams.

The cinema and psychoanalysis have a natural affinity. Claude Chabrol, the esteemed French film-maker, reported in an interview that he had collaborated with a psychoanalyst in the writing of his film, *La Cérémonie* (Feinstein, 1996). He explained why such collaboration was useful: 'It's very hard, when you deal with characters, not to use the Freudian grid, because the Freudian grid is composed of signs that also apply to the cinema' (1996, p. 82).

The marriage between movies and psychoanalysis occurred *in spite of* Sigmund Freud. As far as we know, Freud had little regard for the cinema as an art form and appeared almost oblivious to the development of movies during his lifetime (Sklarew, 1999). His attitude was perhaps best illustrated when Hollywood producer Samuel Goldwyn offered him a $100,000 fee to consult on a film he was planning to shoot in 1925. Freud rejected the offer without a second thought. The *New York Times* of 24 January 1925 displayed the following headline: 'Freud Rebuffs Goldwin: Viennese Psychoanalyst Is Not Interested in Motion Picture Offer' (Sklarew, 1999, p. 1244).

Freud's views were not endorsed by all of his disciples, however. The Austrian director G. W. Pabst sought psychoanalytic consultation when he made his 1926 classic film, *Secrets of a Soul.* He was able to enlist the help of Karl Abraham and Hanns Sachs as psychoanalytic advisers. A psychoanalyst is instrumental to the plot of the film in that he cures the protagonist's knife phobia and impotence through the interpretation of dreams. Indeed, the classic mechanisms of Freud's dreamwork (displacement, condensation and symbolic representation) are depicted with remarkable accuracy.

From the nineteen fifties onwards, analysts began observing that the psychological study of cinematic art might be just as fruitful as Freud's applications of analytic thinking to the plays of Ibsen, Shakespeare and Sophocles (Wolfenstein & Leites, 1950). In subsequent years an entire field of psychoanalytic film criticism has evolved, much of it centred in academic film departments. The French periodical, *Cahiers du Cinéma*, has been extraordinarily influential since it began systematic examinations of American and European films in the nineteen fifties. The *Cahiers* theorists subsequently appropriated Italian semiotics as well as the ideas of the deconstructionist Jacques Derrida and the French psychoanalyst Jacques Lacan. Many of these ideas crossed the Channel and began appearing in the British journal *Screen*, and within a few years American scholars began appropriating the same concepts, especially the psychoanalytically informed feminist critics who wrote for journals such as *Camera Obscura* and *Discourse*.

In 1997 the editorial board of the *International Journal of Psychoanalysis* decided that the time had come to include film reviews alongside the usual collection of book reviews in the pages of the *Journal*. This editorial decision represented an acknowledgement that cinematic art should now be taken seriously as a cultural achievement alongside art, literature, music and drama. Indeed, films have become a storehouse for the psychological images of our time. To a large extent they serve the same functions for contemporary audiences as tragedy served for fifth-century Greeks (Gabbard & Gabbard, 1999). They provide catharsis in a way that is analogous to Greek tragedy, and they also unite audiences with their culture through their mythological dimensions in the same way that Aeschylus or Sophocles provided a vision for the citizens of Athens.

This volume contains a collection of outstanding examples of psychoanalytic film criticism drawn from the first four years of the film review section in the *International Journal of Psychoanalysis* during my tenure as film review editor. Some contributors are academic film scholars, while others are psychoanalysts with a keen interest in film. A number of different theoretical orientations are applied in the film essays contained in this volume, so

the reader will note the same theoretical pluralism that is charac-
teristic of our era's clinical psychoanalysis.

Regardless of one's chosen theoretical orientation to the understanding of film, a set of methodological problems typical of all
applied psychoanalysis must be addressed. First, in the absence of
the associations of a patient and the here-and-now phenomena of
transference and resistance, the psychoanalytically informed film
critic must be creative in identifying material for analysis. Freud
encountered these same difficulties in his forays into applied analysis. In his essay, *Moses and Monotheism*, he made the following
observation: 'I am exposing myself to serious methodological criticism and weakening the convincing force of my arguments. But
this is the only way in which one could treat material of which one
knows definitely that its trustworthiness has been severely
impaired by the distorting influence of tendentious purposes. It is
to be hoped that I shall find some degree of justification later on,
when I come upon the track of these secret motives. Certainty is in
any case unattainable, and moreover, it may be said that every other
writer on the subject has adopted the same procedure' (1939,
p. 27fn.).

Much of the controversy in applied analysis has revolved
around whether the art object itself is the appropriate subject for
analysis, or, rather, the biographical features of the artist that may
contribute to our understanding of the forces shaping the artistic
creation. Both may be fruitful subjects for exploration, and
psychoanalytic film scholars have made productive use of both
approaches. Obviously, when one applies a psychoanalytic lens to
the text of a film, one cannot hope for a definitive reading. A more

modest goal is to emphasise how clinical psychoanalytic theory can illuminate what appears to be happening on the screen and the manner in which the audience experiences it. As Coltrera (1981) has argued in considering applications of psychoanalytic thinking to biography, the primary aims are to be internally consistent and psychoanalytically valid rather than to construct absolute truth. Over time a variety of methodologies have attained some degree of legitimacy as psychoanalytic approaches to film. There are at least seven time-honoured methodological approaches, most of which are illustrated in this volume of psychoanalytic film criticism essays. A brief overview of these prevailing methodologies may help orient the reader to what follows.

THE EXPLICATION OF UNDERLYING CULTURAL MYTHOLOGY

Ray (1985) has stressed that the early Hollywood producers unwittingly served as cultural anthropologists. Their films, especially those that were successful at the box office, tapped into the commonly held unconscious wishes and fears in the mass audience. In pleasing the audience, film-makers also articulate the cultural mythology of the era, specifically Lévi-Strauss's (1975) notion that myths are transformations of fundamental conflicts or contradictions that in reality cannot be resolved. Just as dreams function as wish-fulfilments (at least in many cases), so do films provide wish-fulfilling solutions to human dilemmas. In the 1946 classic, Frank Capra's *It's a Wonderful Life*, for example, the post-World War II audience vicariously experienced the magical resolution of three pervasive internal conflicts: adventure/domesticity, individual/

community and worldly success/ordinary life. As Ray (1985) has argued, the film does not so much resolve these anxieties as push them to one side: George Bailey (James Stewart) joyously declares that money is not important at the same time that friends save his life by showering him with money. *It's a Wonderful Life* strikingly acknowledges its anxieties (as well as those of the culture) in George's fantasy sequence, where a world emerges whole from the darker American visions of *film noir*. Audiences loved Capra's film, however, because its ending so completely disposed of what had briefly returned from the repressed.

In this volume Ronald Baker's essay on the films of Clint Eastwood examines our cultural mythology of screen masculinity. In a thoughtful analysis of *Play 'Misty' for Me*, *Tightrope*, *Unforgiven* and *The Bridges of Madison County*, Baker notes that Clint Eastwood systematically deconstructs the Hollywood myth about what it means to be male, a myth that Eastwood's early films were instrumental in generating. As Baker notes, 'The traditional Hollywood myth of masculinity is thus challenged and undone by the icon of the screen patriarchy himself' (p. 158).

THE FILM AS REFLECTIVE OF THE FILM-MAKER'S SUBJECTIVITY

Biographical material about the *auteur* (the film-maker who is the guiding creative spirit behind a particular film) may shed light on the events and meanings of a particular movie. For example, the extensive hostility towards women documented in Alfred Hitchcock's biographies may help audiences understand the sado-masochistic overtones in male–female relationships in a considerable number of Hitchcock's films (Gabbard, 1998). This biographical material, however, can be submitted to alternative readings as well. Modleski (1988), for example, has used details from Hitchcock's life to argue that the director actually *identified* with women, even placing his male characters in abject, 'feminised' positions comparable to those in which he may have found himself.

This mining of the film-maker's subjectivity to understand a film is illustrated by Argentieri's essay on Truffaut in this collection. She applies a psychoanalytic lens to two of Truffaut's films from the late nineteen seventies, *L'homme qui aimait les femmes* (*The Man Who Loved Women*, 1977) and *La chambre verte* (*The Green Room*, 1978). Argentieri regards these two works as perhaps serving a reparative function for Truffaut. In these films she postulates that Truffaut describes for the audience and for himself his own childhood trauma of not having possessed a symbolic space in the internal world of his mother or the possibility of constructing within himself a safe and stable image of the female figure. These films are thus a canvas in which the director attempts to work through and repair problematic childhood experiences and conflicts.

THE FILM AS REFLECTIVE OF A UNIVERSAL DEVELOPMENTAL MOMENT OR CRISIS

Often the atmosphere or narrative of a film beautifully captures common developmental crises that are vicariously experienced by audience members. For example, one possible reading of Cocteau's 1946 masterpiece, *Beauty and the Beast*, is to view it as a story of an adolescent girl successfully coming to grips with male genitality. In

Ridley Scott's 1979 science fiction film, *Alien*, a paranoid-schizoid
world right out of Melanie Klein is created in which a persecutory
object (the alien) is introjected, reprojected and then is at large
within the space vessel, serving as a source of extraordinary paranoid anxieties (Gabbard & Gabbard, 1999). Part of the appeal of the
horror and science fiction genres is related to the audience's vicarious mastery of infantile anxieties associated with earlier developmental crises. The audience can re-encounter terrifying moments
involving early anxieties while keeping a safe distance from them
and knowing that they can survive them.

The contribution in this volume by noted film scholar Slavoj
Zizek examines both *Titanic* and *Deep Impact* from the perspective
of the Oedipus complex. Zizek suggests that Mimi Leder's *Deep
Impact* (1998), for example, is a drama about an 'unresolved proto-
incestuous father–daughter relationship' (p. 165). Much is made in
the film of how a television reporter (Tea Leoni) is furious at her
father (Maximilian Schell) for divorcing her mother and marrying
a woman the age of his daughter. In this regard, the comet that
threatens to destroy the earth, as seen by Zizek, is related to the
daughter's rage in response to a libidinal catastrophe that has
occurred—namely, her father has chosen another woman over her,
particularly a woman who is approximately her age.

THE APPLICATION OF FREUD'S DREAMWORK TO FILM

Certain films defy conventional analysis and understanding
unless they are viewed as dreams subject to condensation, displacement and other elements of Freud's dreamwork. A consider-

able body of psychoanalytic film criticism has developed around the relationship between film and the 'dream screen', including the work of Kawin (1978), Kinder (1980) and Everwein (1984). The avant-garde film-maker Maya Deren made films that are *only* comprehensible as dreams, and Penley (1989) has suggested that the works of other avant-garde film-makers demand a psychoanalytic reading based on dream theory.

Robert Altman once noted that his 1977 film *Three Women* came to him in a dream (Gabbard & Gabbard, 1999). In fact, if one attempts to approach his movie on a secondary-process level involving rational thinking and coherent narrative style, frustration will ensue. On the other hand, the film becomes comprehensible when viewed at the level of condensation, displacement, symbolisation, dramatisation and the mobile cathexes of the dreamwork described by Freud (1900), Sharpe (1937) and others.

THE ANALYSIS OF SPECTATORSHIP

Film scholars writing from the perspective of Lacan and Derrida focus on the 'deep structures' at work in films and how meaning is generated in the cinema. In so doing, they have placed heavy emphasis on the perspective of the 'spectator' or audience member. Lacan's most important student in the field of film theory has been Metz (1982), whose work has become standard reading in academic film studies courses. The Lacanian approach to film criticism centres on how the perspective of the camera creates a 'gaze' on the events of the film's narrative.

For many years now, the most influential theories of spectatorship have been based in feminist semiotician Laura Mulvey's
'Visual pleasure and narrative cinema' (1975), which appropriated
the concept of 'lack' from Lacanian discourse and suggested that
the woman's body is fetishised in film because it produces anxiety
in the male viewer, to whom the female body represents castration.
Virtually every sentence of this essay has been contested, however,
provoking some of the most important work in the field of psychoanalytic film study. Mulvey herself has rethought her theory
(1989), as have De Lauretis (1984), Hansen (1986), Studlar (1988),
Williams (1989) and Clover (1992). Lacanian analysis of film has
generated considerable criticism in some quarters because the
methodology is regarded as too top-heavy with abstract theoretical
formulations and too focused on the processes through which film
generates meaning rather than the specific content of a given film.
Many psychoanalytic film scholars find the Lacanian approach too
limiting in its insistence on castration, fetishisation and the perspective of a narrowly construed male spectator. Nevertheless,
Lacan continues to inspire some of the most important film theorists, most notably Slavoj Zizek (1992) and Joan Copjec (1995).

The semiotic theories of spectatorship have spawned a greater
awareness of the interplay between a film and its audience. A
good deal of recent psychoanalytic film criticism is based on the
notion that specific assumptions in the spectator interact with
the visual aspects of a film and its narrative to illuminate particular psychoanalytically informed meanings. My own essay on *The
Crying Game* in this volume is emblematic of this approach, while
also drawing on some universal developmental themes.

THE APPROPRIATION OF
PSYCHOANALYTIC CONSTRUCTS BY THE FILM-MAKER

Yet another methodological approach is to examine how certain psychoanalytic constructs (e.g. splitting, repression, displacement, condensation) are utilised (often unconsciously) by the director, cinematographer or screenwriter to make a particular point. Cinematic techniques appropriating free association or primary process may make a specific visual montage more psychologically true to the viewer. Content may also corroborate analytic ideas. The psychoanalytic notion that memories are inevitably filtered through the subjectivity of the individual, for example, is the centrepiece of Kurosawa's *Rashomon* (1950). Raoul Walsh's western, *Pursued*, was using psychoanalytically based flashback narration as early as 1947.

Indeed, it is striking to note the extent to which psychoanalytic ideas have infiltrated the American cinema. Even in a mainstream 'popcorn' movie like Jan de Bont's 1996 *Twister*, psychoanalytic ideas are central to the narrative form. Helen Hunt, the protagonist in *Twister*, plays a scientist who chases tornadoes with a fervour that seems driven by unconscious forces. Through a flashback the audience learns early on that the Helen Hunt character lost her father to a tornado when she was a child. Hence, the drivenness is explained by the familiar psychoanalytic construct of active mastery over passively experienced trauma. In her efforts to master the mysteries of tornadoes, she will somehow overcome her childhood trauma and work through her grief at the loss of her father.

THE ANALYSIS OF A CHARACTER IN THE NARRATIVE

This approach of applying psychoanalytic understanding to illuminate the motives of a character has fallen out of favour in recent years among psychoanalytic film critics. Greater emphasis is now placed on the *function* of a character or the film-maker's overarching purpose rather than the motivations of the character. Some argue that characters in film are not, in fact, real, and therefore analysis is misguided and doomed to failure from the outset. Nevertheless, Freud employed such methodology with impressive results when he examined the character of Rebecca in Ibsen's play *Rosmersholm* (1916). Freud did not explain, however, how Ibsen was able to create a character who yielded her mysteries so completely to psychoanalysis. Of course, Ibsen was a scrupulous observer of human pathology, and Freud was a brilliant reader of literary texts. Anyone writing on film today must be able to explain how a film-maker constructs a character that seems to emerge full-blown from a case history.

In this collection of essays Jacob Arlow's perspective on Izak Borg in Bergman's *Wild Strawberries* has much in common with Freud's analysis of Rebecca in *Rosmersholm*. He finds meaning to be gleaned in the dreams of Borg as though they were the dreams of a patient. He also plumbs the depths of Borg's unconscious to shed light on universal psychological struggles involving time and ageing.

CONCLUDING COMMENTS

These diverse methodologies obviously overlap to some extent in many analyses of film. Some psychoanalytic film critics deliberately mix methodologies for a more comprehensive reading of a particular text. In Adrienne Harris's chapter on the Quentin Tarentino film *Reservoir Dogs* (1991), she ingeniously melds different approaches to support her reading of the film as an expression of the ungrieved and lingering trauma of Vietnam in American consciousness. Harris describes her methodology as follows: 'I am using here a mixed model drawing on an evolving feminist theory (Penley, 1989), reception theory, which is a psychoanalytically driven theory of how meaning is evolved and managed (Zizek, 1994), and a psychoanalytic reading of film as the expression of underlying, often unconscious cultural tensions and contradictions' (pp. 75-6).

The psychoanalytic methodologies are separated out here for the purpose of illustrating the diversity of methodological approaches inherent in applied psychoanalysis of film. The true test of any of these approaches is the extent to which the reader views the film under consideration from a new and enlightening point of view, which often requires examining the film from a variety of perspectives. In a penetrating contribution on the application of psychoanalytic thinking to artistic creations, Kaplan noted, 'A psychoanalytic reflection on any phenomenon is incisive to the extent that it employs more than one dimension. This is why ... the analogy of Ahab's quest for his mother in the guise of Moby Dick falls short of anything really worth saying psychoanalytically' (1988, p. 283).

The fundamental psychoanalytic notion of multiple determination has been applied to a variety of cinematic texts. Among the leading exemplars of this multi-dimensional approach are Cavell

(1981), Wood (1986), Ray (1985), and Gabbard & Gabbard (1999).
A multiplicity of theoretical perspectives is brought to bear in these
different approaches, and the result is a psychoanalytic film criticism that understands a particular movie as having multi-layered
meanings that are not immediately apparent to the average viewer.

To conclude, audiences do not attend films merely to be enter-
tained. They line up at the local multiplex to encounter long-for-
gotten but still powerful anxieties that stem from universal
developmental experiences. They seek solutions to problems in the
culture that defy simple answers or facile explanations. The screen
in the darkened theatre serves as a container for the projection of
their most private and often unconscious terrors and longings. As
with all forms of art, when we study film we study ourselves.

REFERENCES

CAVELL, S. (1981). *Pursuits of Happiness: The Hollywood Comedy of Remarriage.* Cambridge, MA: Harvard Univ. Press.

CLOVER, C. (1992). *Men, Women and Chainsaws.* Princeton, NJ: Princeton Univ. Press

COLTRERA, J. T. (1981). *Pursuits of Happiness: The Hollywood Comedy of Remarriage.* Cambridge, MA: Harvard Univ. Press.

COPJEC, J. (1995). *Read My Desire: Lacan Against the Historicists.* Cambridge, MA: MIT Press.

DE LAURETIS, T. (1984). *Alice Doesn't: Feminism, Semiotics, Cinema.* Bloomington, IN: Indiana Univ. Press.

EHRENBURG, I. (1931). *Die Traumfabriki Chronik des Films.* Berlin: Malik.

EVERWEIN, R. E. (1984). *Film and the Dream Screen*. Princeton, NJ: Princeton Univ. Press

FEINSTEIN, H. (1996). Killer instincts: director Claude Chabrol finds madness in his method. *Village Voice*, 24 December 1996, p. 86.

FREUD, S. (1900). *The Interpretation of Dreams. S.E.* 4-5.

—— (1939). *Moses and Monotheism: Three Essays. S.E.* 23.

GABBARD, G. O. (1998). *Vertigo*: Female objectification, male desire, and object loss. *Psychoanal. Inq.*, 18: 161-167.

GABBARD, K. & GABBARD G. O. (1999). *Psychiatry and the Cinema: 2nd Edition*. Washington, DC: American Psychiatric Press.

HANSEN, M. (1986). Pleasure, ambivalence, identification: Valentino and female spectatorship. *Cinema Journal*, 25: 6-32.

KAPLAN, D. M. (1988). The psychoanalysis of art: some ends, some means. *J. Amer. Psychoanal. Assn.*, 36: 259-93.

KAWIN, B. (1978) *Mindscreen: Bergaman, Godard, and First-Person Film*. Princeton, NJ: Princeton Univ. Press.

KINDER, M. (1980). The adaptation of cinematic dreams. *Dreamworks*, 1: 51-68.

LEVI-STRAUSS, C. (1975). *The Raw and the Cooked: Introduction to a Science of Mythology: I*. Trans. J. and D. Weightman. New York: Harper & Row.

METZ, C. (1982). *The Imaginary Signifier: Psychoanalysis and the Cinema*, trans. C. Britton et al. Bloomington, IN: Indiana Univ. Press.

MODLESKI, T. (1988). *The Women Who Knew Too Much: Hitchcock and Feminist Theory*. New York: Methuen.

MULVEY, L. (1975). Visual pleasure and narrative cinema. *Screen*, 16: 61-18.

—— (1989). *Visual and Other Pleasures.* Bloomington, IN: Indiana Univ. Press.

MÜNSTERBERG, H. (1916). *The Film: A Psychological Study.* New York: Dover, 1970.

PENLEY, C. (1989). *Feminism and Film Theory.* New York: Routledge.

RAY, R. B. (1985). *A Certain Tendency of the Hollywood Cinema, 1930-1980.* Princeton, NJ: Princeton Univ. Press.

SCHNEIDER, I. (1985). The psychiatrist in the movies: the first 50 years. In *The Psychoanalytic Study of Literature,* ed. J. Reppen & M. Charney. Hillsdale, NJ: Analytic Press, pp. 53–67.

SHARPE, E. (1937). *Dream Analysis.* New York: Brunner/Mazel.

SKLAREW, B. (1999). Freud and film: encounters in the *weltgeist. J. Amer. Pyschoanal. Assn.,* 47: 1239-1247.

STUDLAR, G. (1988). *In the Realm of Pleasure: Von Steernberg, Dietrich and the Masochistic Aesthetic.* Urbana, IL: Univ. of Illinois Press.

WILLIAMS, L. (1989). *Hard Core: Power, Pleasure, and the Frenzy of the Visible.* Berkeley, CA: Univ. of California Press.

WOLFENSTEIN, M. & LEITES, N. (1950). *Movies: A Psychological Study.* Glencoe, IL: Free Press.

WOOD, R. (1986). *Hollywood Film from Vietnam to Reagan.* New York: Columbia Univ. Press.

ZIZEK, S. (ED.) (1992). *Everything You Always Wanted to Know About Lacan (But Were Afraid to Ask Hitchcock).* New York: Verso.

—— (1994). *The Metastases of Enjoyment.* London: Verso.

2. THE END OF TIME:
A PSYCHOANALYTIC PERSPECTIVE ON INGMAR BERGMAN'S *WILD STRAWBERRIES*

JACOB A. ARLOW, KING'S POINT, NY

On the morning of a special day, the day he is to receive an honorary doctorate for his contributions to humanity and science, Dr Izak Borg awakens from an unusual and disturbing dream. He is a testy old man of 75, a widower, with a surviving mother of 95, and a son, Ewald, like himself a physician. As *Wild Strawberries*, Ingmar Bergman's classic masterpiece, unfolds, through dreams, reminiscences and the events of that single day, we come to know and understand the central character with a penetrating insight, the kind that, as a rule, comes only from long and arduous psychoanalytic treatment. Accordingly, this film should hold a special enchantment for psychoanalysts.

In the dream, Dr Borg finds himself in a strange and unfamiliar neighbourhood, devoid of any sign of life. He looks up at a street clock. It has no hands. From his pocket he pulls a watch, a junior version of the larger clock. It too has no hands. All around there is dead silence, but at that moment we begin to hear the beating of Izak's heart. (For a clock without hands, time does not move. Izak is in the realm of timeless eternity, i.e. death.) Bewildered, Izak looks about and sees a man standing with his back to him. As he touches him, the man turns slightly, his face swathed in gauze-like bandages, obliterating his features.

The figure topples over and the head falls away from the body as blood gushes from the neck into a small pool. (In effect, Izak has killed a dead man.) At that moment the silence is broken by the tolling of church bells, while around the bend in the street comes a hearse drawn by two horses but with no rider. As the hearse proceeds past Izak, one of the rear wheels gets caught in a lamppost. The hearse thrusts forward, thrusts forward again and again, until the wheel, freed from its attachment, rolls back at great speed, barely missing Izak. In the process, the hearse tilts over, expelling the coffin it had held. As Izak approaches the coffin, the corpse grasps his hand, pulling him closer. To his consternation, Izak sees that the face of the corpse is his own. He awakens, deeply disturbed.

What Izak does next is striking. Although it is still early in the morning, he bursts into the room of Miss Agda, his long-time housekeeper, and wakes her with his decision to alter their travel plans. Instead of taking the plane to Malmö, where his son will be waiting for him, he intends to drive directly to Lund, although it means he will be arriving much later than planned. (Unconsciously, he is behaving like the servant in O'Hara's parable, *Appointment in Samara*, who had hoped to escape the Angel of Death by changing the time and the place of their presumably ordained encounter. This manoeuvre parallels Freud's interpretation of the typical dream of missing a train, namely, the wish not to be 'there' at the appointed hour of death. The one who determines the time and place of the appointment is the master of life and death.)[1]

---

[1] A similar dynamic often applies to who controls the time of the psychoanalytic appointment.

Marianne, Izak's daughter-in-law, who has been staying at his
home because of some differences with her husband, volunteers to
accompany him on the long journey to Lund. On the way we
observe more of Dr Borg's unpleasant character, although a gentle
wistfulness seems to break through from time to time. Miss Agda
has already labelled him a selfish old man but, in addition, we learn
that he is demeaning and hostile towards women. Smoking, for
example, is a pleasure to be reserved for men. Women may indulge
themselves, if they wish, in such pleasures as crying, caring for children and gossiping. If the troubles between Marianne and Ewald
are financial, Izak is of no mind to forgive the debt they owe him. If
the difficulties are emotional, he suggests she go to a priest or to
some quack psychologist.

On the way he makes a detour to the vacation house where his
family spent the first twenty summers of his life. They were ten
brothers and sisters, but he is the only one who has survived. He
wants to tell Marianne about it but she is not interested. She goes
for a swim, while Izak seats himself on the ground near the old wild
strawberry patch and, in a visual memory, recalls the events of
another special day, his father's birthday. Izak's beautiful cousin,
Sara, is in the wild strawberry patch picking the fruit, a birthday
gift for her uncle. Sara and Izak are in love and they have an understanding to be married. In his reverie, Izak sees how his next
younger brother, Sigfrid, comes upon Sara and makes advances
towards her, all the while belittling Izak as a weakling. In the end,
Sara succumbs to his seduction.

In the next scene the family is assembled at the birthday table
while Izak, the old man, is the unseen onlooker. Mother is an over-

bearing martinet, putting everyone down. Father is a ludicrous figure, floppy moustache, stone-deaf, sporting a ridiculous hearing aid
which clearly does no good. While father is receiving the gifts, the
obnoxious girl twins reveal how they saw Sara and Sigfrid having a
tryst in the wild strawberry patch. Humiliated and in tears, Sara
flees the table to an adjoining room where she is comforted by a
female relative. There she confesses that, although Izak is kind, sensitive, generous, spiritual, high-minded and poetic, nevertheless she
feels sometimes that she is older than him and thinks of him as a
little boy. Sigfrid, on the other hand, is wild and exciting, forward
and aggressive. She makes it clear it is child versus man.

Two things are noteworthy at this point. First the choice of
names. Izak, i.e. Isaac, stems from Christian scripture. The biblical
Isaac is gentle and submissive, even ready to serve as a sacrificial
animal for his father, Abraham. Sigfrid, on the other hand, stems
from the bold, aggressive Norse-German tradition. More significant, however, is Sara's description of Izak's character at the time of
the wild strawberry patch trauma. Instead of the demeaning, insen-
sitive, selfish person in the car on the road to Lund, he had once
been a gentle, sensitive young man. It is as if Izak had become a
caricature of Sigfrid, cruel and self-centred, exaggerating the latter's worst traits. In the transformation of his character, Izak seems
to be saying to Sara, 'If that's the kind of man you prefer, that's the
kind of person I will be. Even more so'. In part, his vengeance takes
the form of an identification with the aggressor, but sadly such
transformations can easily give way to self-loathing and self-hatred.

Izak is roused from his reverie by the voice of a young girl. She is
saucy and seductive, secure in the knowledge of her beauty and rev-

elling in its exercise. A mild but definite flirtation develops between them. She says, 'My name is Sara, a rotten name'. He says, 'My name is Izak, rotten too'. She asks, 'Weren't they a couple?' 'No', he says, 'that was Abraham and Sarah'. (The young girl's 'mistake' of memory subtly but definitely introduces the incest motif. Sarah and Isaac were mother and son.) The flirtation now continues on Izak's part. He says, 'A girl I loved when I was young was also named Sara'. 'Was she like me?' 'Well, to tell the truth, she was quite like you.' 'What happened to her later?' 'She married my younger brother, Sigfrid, and had six boys. Now she is 75 years old and rather a beautiful woman.'

Young Sara, with two boyfriends in tow, is on her way to Italy, and Izak and Marianne give them a hitch. In the car, high-spirited and forward, Sara engages Izak with the details of her love life. She is engaged to one of the boys who is sweet and idealistic, preparing to be a minister, but at the same time, she says, she is trying to seduce the other, who is bold and practical, preparing to be a scientist. Of course, she says, she can behave this way because she is still a virgin. This recapitulation of the Izak-Sigfrid rivalry is played out throughout the rest of the film. In fact, at one point the two rivals for young Sara actually come to blows.

At this point in the trip there is a near-accident. A car, driving in the opposite direction and in the wrong lane, swerves sharply off the road and, reminiscent of the hearse in the opening dream, turns over. Because she had been quarrelling with her husband, the wife of the couple lost control of the car. She was about to strike her husband. The man, apologetically yet in a most demeaning and insulting way, blames the accident on his wife. Marianne offers the couple a lift. In the car, they continue unabashedly their sado-maso-chistic assault upon each other, to the astonished and stunned disbelief of the young people watching in the back. It becomes too much for Marianne, who asks the couple to leave because she does not want to expose the young people to so abhorrent a scene.

The primal scene element so clearly depicted in this incident has in fact already been adumbrated several times earlier in the course of the film. First was the repetitive thrusting of the hearse against the lamppost in the initial dream. Next was Izak's intrusion into Miss Agda's bedroom, awakening her from her sleep while she modestly clasped the bedclothes about her. Then came Marianne's experience of being disturbed by the noise of the quarrel between Izak and Miss Agda at the breakfast table and, finally and unmistakably, Izak's re-viewing in his mind the seduction in the wild strawberry patch that the obnoxious twins had observed.

Driving through the region where Dr Borg first began his practice and where his old mother lives, he stops at a gas station to refill his tank. The owner recalls Izak's many kindnesses and, out of gratitude, refuses to accept payment for the fuel. Reluctantly, Dr Borg accepts the gift but asks to be sent a note when the pregnant wife of the gas station owner delivers. He insists upon being the godfather of the new child. Leaving the young people at the lunch table, Izak and Marianne go to visit the elderly Mrs Borg. Clearly her mental powers have deteriorated. She mistakes Marianne for Izak's wife. Izak reminds his mother that his wife is dead and that this is Ewald's wife, to which the mother says to Marianne, 'Why aren't you home tending your children?' and she adds that she had ten children. 'They are all dead except Izak.' The irony here is profound since all of Izak's rivals, oedipal and pre-oedipal, father, Sigfrid, the nasty twins and the rest are all gone. Now he alone is left with the two women whom at one time or another in his life he had wanted most of all, but it is all empty and meaningless.

The mother is reviewing mementos from her child-rearing years; a doll belonging to one of Izak's sisters, a picture of Sigfrid and Izak when they were 3 and 5, a little book in which one of the sisters wrote: 'Most of all in the world I love Papa', and the other added, 'I'm going to marry Papa'. Izak's mother then comes upon the father's watch. She had been thinking of giving it to Sigfrid's older son, who is going to be 50 soon. She asks, 'Can I give it to him, even though the hands are off?' It is the very watch without hands which Izak saw in the opening dream and, as he looks at it, once again we hear the beating of his heart. As if to add insult to injury, the mother adds, 'I remember when Sigfrid's baby was born and lying in his cradle. Now he will be 50 years old and little cousin Sara always cradled him and lulled him to sleep. She married Sigfrid, that good-for-nothing'.

As they resume their journey, Izak falls asleep once again and is haunted by dreams and visions, at once overpowering and humiliating. 'Something that penetrated deep into my consciousness with almost unbearable determination.'[2]

In the dream, once again Izak is in the wild strawberry patch. Cousin Sara is saying to him, 'Have you looked in the mirror? I will

[2] This long, revealing and interesting dream, unfortunately, cannot be described or discussed fully, given the limitations of space for this presentation.

show you how you look. You are a frightened old man who will soon
die and I have my life ahead of me. I am sorry if I have offended you'.
Nonetheless, she continues to taunt him, calling attention to his
pain, to his ignorance and, in an ultimate bit of cruelty, she tells him,
'I must go now. I promised to look after Sigfrid's little boy'.

In the next sequence of the dream, Izak is outside the house,
looking through the window at Sara and Sigfrid in loving relationship. She plays the piano and he caresses her tenderly. Then they go
to a table and have drinks together. Suddenly the lights go out, the
door opens and the man whom we shall call 'the Examiner' appears.
He leads Izak through long, dark corridors (of memory?) to the
examination room. Barely visible, seated in a small gallery like a
jury box, immobile and expressionless, are young Sara and her two
friends with another person, possibly Marianne. Izak is asked to
look into the microscope and to identify the bacteria. Izak says he
sees nothing (i.e. he cannot see the cause of the illness). He is asked
to read the handwriting on the blackboard but he doesn't know
what it means. 'The message', the Examiner says, 'is a doctor's first
professional duty. What is it?' Izak can't recall. The Examiner says,
'The doctor's first professional duty is to beg for forgiveness'. 'Ah,
yes', says Izak, 'I remember now'. Izak is asked whether he pleads
guilty or not guilty, but he doesn't understand. He protests, 'I am an
old man. Spare me'. Izak is then asked to do an anamnesis and examine a woman patient. 'But the patient is dead', Izak protests. There-
upon the patient, who is his wife, begins to laugh. The joke is on
Izak. (Once again he refuses to review the history which would
explain the cause of the trouble.) The verdict of the Examiner is that
Izak is incompetent and he says, 'Moreover, you have been accused

of smaller, but nonetheless serious crimes; indifference, selfishness, lack of consideration'. The accusations have been made by his wife, the Examiner says, and now they will confront her. 'She has been dead for many years', protests Izak, but the Examiner now invites him to confront his past.

Like Virgil demonstrating to Dante the torments of hell, the Examiner leads Izak to a garden, to a scene that he experienced on a specific date in his life. Izak observes his wife in an act of adultery. It is clear that she has been driven to this by his indifference. Adjusting her clothes after having had intercourse, she says that she will go home and confess her adultery to Izak. She will ask to be forgiven but he will say there is nothing to be forgiven. He didn't care enough to be offended; he had been killing her with kindness.

Suddenly the garden is empty. 'Where is she?' Izak asks. 'She is gone. All are gone. Everything has been removed.' 'What is the penalty?' Izak asks. 'The usual one, I suppose', says the Examiner, 'loneliness', and at this point Izak awakens from his dream. He tells his daughter-in-law that he has been dreaming about things that he couldn't quite tell himself when he was awake, i.e. what he doesn't want to hear is that he is already dead, even though he is still alive. It is then that the daughter-in-law reveals that her husband, Izak's son Ewald, says the same thing. Even though he is only 38, he feels that he is old and dead.

The conflict between Marianne and her husband is over having a child. He doesn't want one and she does. He is another edition of his father—cruel, cold and rational. He believes it is absurd to add new victims to this cruel world. He himself was an unwanted child in an unhappy marriage. Later Izak affirms that this was so, and he notes that the scene of the couple fighting in his car was a reminder of his own marriage. Finally the time arrives for the bestowing of the honorary doctorate. Solemn and austere, the academic procession reminds one above all of a funeral. There are only men in the line of march, all dressed in black. The initiates, Dr Borg among them, are bareheaded while those who escort them all wear black top hats. The procession is made up entirely of men, the audience entirely of women. Dr Izak Borg ascends the podium, standing erect and impassive, while the installer, like some primitive tribal chief, chants the incomprehensible and untranslated Latin and ends by placing the black top hat on Izak's head.[3]

Two very touching scenes close the film. Izak hears singing under the window. The young people have come to serenade him. Young Sara says that he was fantastic in the parade and they were so proud of him, but now they are leaving. 'We came to say goodbye. Goodbye, Father Izak', she says, 'you are the one I really love, today, tomorrow and forever'. He says, 'I'll remember that', and then, when they are probably out of earshot, he says, 'Let's hear from you sometime', although deep down he must know that he probably never will and, even if he did, what of it? The problem is time, time that is always out of joint, time, the eternal frustrator: in childhood, because we are powerless and lack authority; in old age, because we no longer have the opportunity.

As the film closes, Izak makes two desperate attempts to repair the past. He offers to be more friendly to Miss Agda, but she will

[3] Shortly before his death, Henry Alden Bunker said to me that death is the final initiation, the ultimate marker of manhood.

have none of it. He wants to alleviate the tension between his son and Marianne, but as he begins to offer to forgive the debt they owe him, before he can finish, Ewald cuts him off and tells him not to be concerned, the debt will be repaid. No repair has accrued from his belated insight. The past cannot be undone. Once again his thoughts turn to the events of his youth and he hears Sara saying, 'Izak, there are no strawberries left'. With mixed nostalgia and regret, Izak turns in his bed and goes to sleep.

'For of all sad words of tongue or pen,

The saddest are these: it might have been.'

John Greenleaf Whittier.

3. HITCHCOCK'S *VERTIGO*: THE COLLAPSE OF A RESCUE FANTASY

EMANUEL BERMAN, ISRAEL

'Just as, in the end, the detective is revealed to be the criminal, the doctor-therapist, the would-be analyst, herself turns out to be but an analysand. *The Turn of the Screw* in fact deconstructs all these traditional oppositions; the exorcist and the possessed, the doctor and the patient, the sickness and the cure, the symptom and the proposed interpretation of the symptom, here become interchangeable, or at the very least, undecidable' (Felman, 1982, p. 176).

This paper offers a psychoanalytic exploration of Alfred Hitchcock's film, *Vertigo* (1958). I will start from my own view of the film, continue with a review of the extensive literature debating it and conclude with a discussion of a few issues related to the way in which *Vertigo* has been understood and of some fundamental dilemmas in the psychoanalytic study of art.

A PERSONAL VIEW

John 'Scottie' Ferguson, the protagonist of *Vertigo*, is a detective haunted by his human frailty: his vertigo. The way in which this film activates audience involvement is a crucial aspect of its power: as viewers, we become deeply identified with Scottie's vulnerability.

We follow him in his heroic but miscarried quest to overcome it. Remembering—when we can—that Scottie and the other figures we watch are actually fictional film characters, we are forced to realise that what we are truly exploring is our own fears, fantasies and identifications as enthralled viewers.

In the opening scene of the film, trauma occurs: we encounter Scottie's impotence (and our own) while his colleague—attempting to rescue him—falls from a roof-top to his death (fig. 1). From now on, Scottie continuously strives to overcome the trauma, to regain mastery, to undo his humiliation. He makes desperate efforts to rescue himself from the chaotic fearful regression constantly lurking behind the brittle shell of his reality.

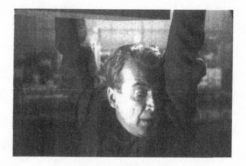

Fig. 1: Scottie's trauma

But consciously, maybe projectively, his quest shifts to the rescue of another person: the enchanting woman we come to know as Madeleine. When asked by Gavin Elster— his college friend, who tells him she is his wife—to help her, he responds by saying: 'Take her to the nearest psychiatrist, or psychologist, or neurologist, or psychoana ... '. He is about to say 'psychoanalyst' but never completes the word. Yet Scottie soon finds himself in the role of a psychoanalyst: searching for Madeleine's lost memories, attempting to interpret her dreams, seeking the integration of dissociated personality fragments, striving to liberate Madeleine from the claws of her enigmatic obsession and free her to live and to love.

I came to realise that Scottie's drama richly resonates with my own experiences as a psychoanalyst. In my imagination he becomes an analyst grappling with his unavoidable deep emotional involvement and unconscious identifications; with the impossibility both of maintaining detached objectivity, and of guaranteeing one's role as a reparative good object or selfobject; with the dangers of grandiosity, of omniscience, of illusory control. In my personal viewing of the film—coloured, naturally, by my own psychic reality—it is a tale of 'transference love' but also of 'countertransference love', that crystallises around a rescue fantasy (fig. 2). Rescuing Madeleine from drowning, Scottie becomes—as many of us are, in our daydreams—Orpheus, struggling to bring Eurydice back from Hades. He takes us along in his quest, graphically depicted in the film as a dangerous spiral descent.

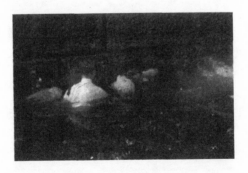

Fig. 2: The rescue concretised

The first part of the film strongly establishes this fantasy, accurately corresponding to its most ancient mythical portrayals. Madeleine is Beauty, captivated and endangered by an obscure, unseen Dragon (fig. 3). Whether this Dragon will turn out to be psychological (neurotic fantasy or childhood experience), metaphysical (the spirit of Madeleine's ancestor Carlotta Valdes, who had been ditched, deprived of her child and driven mad) or criminal (a possibility raised much later in the film), Scottie is willing to fight it: he assumes the role of the Knight, determined to find the Dragon and behead it. At this stage, as in the classical rescue legend, these three key roles are sharply differentiated, through splitting and disavowal, which mask any potential concordant or complementary identifications between the figures. This defensive myth-making necessarily deprives the participants of their conflictual three-dimensionality: the valiant, masterful and selfsacrificing Knight is utterly different from lost, confused and helpless Beauty, and could have nothing in common with the mortal enemy, the vicious Dragon.

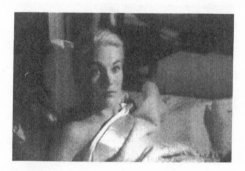

Fig. 3: Madeleine: an obscure object of desire

Naturally, the Knight falls in love with Beauty; the helpless object of rescue and the romantic object of desire merge, and this combination has an enormous impact on the protagonist, and on the viewers identified with his vision. (We are, like Scottie, annoyed with his friend Midge's scepticism and sarcasm towards his credulous fascination.) Scottie is also gradually able to win Madeleine's love, in spite of her reserve and hesitation. After successfully rescuing her from her apparent suicide attempt in the waters of San Francisco Bay, he tells her: 'once you've saved a person's life, you are responsible for them forever'; and then, while reassuring her 'no one possesses you' he also says 'I've got you'. Coming to believe he has distinguished reality from fantasy in her story, and found the clue to the fearful recurrent dream she describes ('it will finish your dream'), as well as to the whole mystery, he is self-assuredly approaching his ultimate victory.

But here we are confronted with the film's first cruel turnabout: at the crucial moment Scottie is incapacitated by his acrophobia and vertigo, cannot follow Madeleine up the bell tower's steep staircase, and rather than fulfilling his and our fantasy wish by rescuing her (and himself) he is confronted with a second traumatic fall, Madeleine's fall to her death—fig. 4 below:

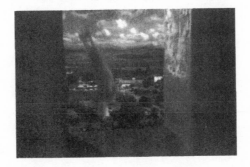

At this horrifying moment the first element of splitting and disavowal in the rescue myth crumbles: we painfully come to realise that
our Knight is as helpless, lonely and desperate as his Beauty. This is
soon underlined by the guilt-enhancing pronouncement of the investigating official, an unrelentingly harsh superego representative, as well
as by Scottie's nightmare, in which he is now the one falling into the
open grave, he is himself beheaded, it is he who is plunging to the roof
below, then into a void. We fully experience now both the yearning to
fall and the terror of falling, combined in vertigo. Yes, 'someone out of
the past, someone dead, can enter and take possession of a living being'.

Hospitalised for his acute melancholia and guilt, Scottie appears for
a while to be overwhelmed by his loss, to be mentally dead, as he
motionlessly defies all rescue attempts, now directed towards him by
Midge and the doctors (fig. 5).

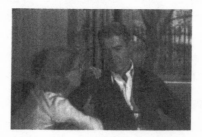

Fig. 5: Scottie motionlessly defies rescue

Eventually discharged, Scottie looks for Madeleine in the streets of
San Francisco, just as Carlotta, Madeleine's unfortunate ancestor,
reportedly looked for her lost daughter (and as Hanold looked for
Gradiva in the streets of Pompeii). He finally appears to discover her in
the person of Judy, a lonely young woman who left home after the death

of her beloved father (fig. 6). While our first guess may be that this is a delusional attempt to undo Madeleine's death, Hitchcock allows us for the first time—in a bold departure from the original book and from the traditions of the genre—to discover the truth that still eludes our protagonist. The flashback scene clarifies reality, but also re-establishes the rescue myth by personalising the Dragon. It was Gavin Elster who killed his actual wife, exploited dressed-up Judy as a decoy, and manipulated Scottie so cruelly in order to use him as a witness to Madeleine's apparent suicide.

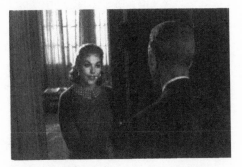

Fig. 6: Judy first encounters Scottie

Now we realise how naïve was Scottie's romanticised view of the situation and of his role. The understanding that he had reached had been so partial that it blinded him to the deeper truth. The further discoveries we make later on make this realisation even more poignant and tragic.

Knowing now the actual history, we are finally allowed to be the insightful analysts, the successful detectives. Aware of Judy's real love for Scottie, and of her moving anguish, both established in the scene in which she writes him a confessional farewell letter but then destroys it and decides to stay, we now abandon our full identification with Scottie. Through the film's conclusion we find ourselves identified with both Scottie and Judy, and therefore in constant conflict between their points of view, and in full awareness of the pain involved in a deep relationship between two individuals with divergent subjectivities. Having no longer a Knight to rely on, we ourselves become the fantasised Knight, wishing to rescue both our vulnerable protagonists from the emotional aftermath of Elster's vicious scheme.

The process is tantalising. Scottie, dominated by a tenacious Pygmalion fantasy, obsessively and fetishistically attempts now to mould Judy into Madeleine, in spite of her reluctance and fear. Fear of being found out, fear of being exploited once more, but also fear of losing her identity, of being forced to maintain permanently the elevated fantasy persona of Madeleine? Eventually, her love for Scottie gains the upper hand, and she abandons her struggle to keep both of them in a 'real' world, in which she would be free to be herself. She succumbs, and agrees to recreate Madeleine fully, to disappear 'under the shadow of (his) object' in order to reach her object. Her reappearance transformed into Madeleine is a breathtaking moment of romantic fantasy fulfilment; Scottie feels he has succeeded in defying death, in bringing Eurydice back from Hades; Judy hopes finally to regain his lasting love. Yet, the illusory brittle fictitiousness of this moment makes it uncanny, scary and ominous (fig. 7 on facing page).

Shortly afterwards comes Orpheus's forbidden look, which will send Eurydice back to hell. Judy absentmindedly wears Carlotta's and Madeleine's necklace—out of an unconscious urge to confess her guilt and atone for it? Because living and loving deceptively is unbearable?

Or because of her longing for the persona of Madeleine, which fulfilled her own potential? (fig. 8).

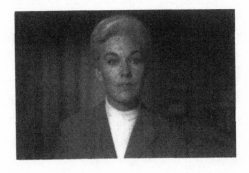

Fig. 7: Judy recreated as Madeleine

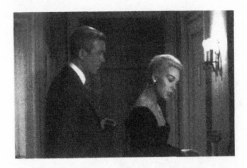

Fig. 8: The Orphean forbidden look

Scottie, in a split second, guesses the truth. And now, in the heart-breaking final scene, the last Maginot-line of splitting and disavowal also falls, and with it the mythical rescue fantasy completely collapses. Scottie comes to see the similarity between him and Gavin Elster, the exact parallel between the two stages of creating and recreating (as film directors do) the fetishistic romantic object, the make-believe phantom figure of Madeleine: 'He made you over just like I made you over'. The woman who was his object of compassion and passion turns out to have been the creation of another man (we are reminded of Nathaniel and Olympia in 'The Sandman'). He now finds himself dragging Judy up the bell-tower's staircase with enraged, ruthless cruelty, almost choking her.

He may be overcoming his vertigo, but he is losing his humanity and the meaning of his life. His identification with the distressed woman has been transformed into sadistic and vengeful domination. In his desperate attempt to find the truth and free himself from a deception by a villain, he has sunk into a deceptive delusion of his own, and gradually turns into the villain. John the Saviour turns out, after all, to be Jack the Ripper. The Knight has become the Dragon (fig. 9 below).

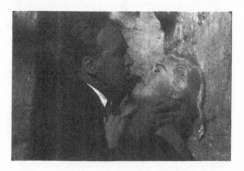

By ultimately destroying the illusory Madeleine, Scottie is also terrifying the real Judy, his flesh-and-blood beloved and loving Beauty. Their
final hug arouses faint hopes of reparation, but the sudden appearance
of a nun at the bell-tower makes Judy stumble and fall to her death. As
we hear the bell, we are reminded of John Donne's lines: 'Now, this Bell
tolling softly for another, saies to me, Thou must die ... No man is an
Iland, intire of it selfe ... And therefore never send to know for whom
the bell tolls; it tolls for thee' (*Devotions*, 1624, xvi-xvii).

A REVIEW OF THE LITERATURE

Perhaps the greatest weakness in the psychoanalytic studies of literature is that they rarely acknowledge that several interpretations may
all plausibly reveal something about a work of art (Werman, 1979, p.
475).

Vertigo is one of the most intensely debated films in the history of
cinema (White, 1991). Although the vast literature analysing it is not
usually written by practising analysts, most of it deals with psychoanalytic issues, being part of a unique trend in contemporary academic
film scholarship, strongly influenced by Freud and Lacan, as well as by
Marx, Althusser and particularly feminist thought (Kaplan, 1990, p. 9).

A central figure within this tradition is Laura Mulvey, who opened
the debate in her 1975 paper, 'Visual pleasure and narrative cinema'.
She interprets Scottie's pursuit of Madeleine as an erotic obsession
based on castration anxiety, stating: 'Scottie's voyeurism is blatant: he
falls in love with a woman he follows and spies on without speaking to.
Its sadistic side is equally blatant ... Once he actually confronts her, his
erotic drive is to break her down and force her to tell by persistent

cross-questioning. Then, in the second part of the film, he re-enacts his obsessive involvement ... He reconstructs Judy as Madeleine, forces her to conform in every detail to the actual physical appearance of his fetish ... in the repetition he does break her down and succeeds in exposing her guilt. His curiosity wins through and she is punished' (Mulvey, 1975, p. 66).

While harshly accusatory towards Scottie, Mulvey judges Judy severely as well: 'Her exhibitionism, her masochism, make her an ideal passive counterpart to Scottie's active sadistic voyeurism' (fig. 10).

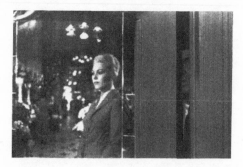

Fig. 10: Voyeurism or identification?

A very different view of the film's dynamics was soon offered by the interrelated works of Spoto (1976, 1983) and Wood (1977, 1989). Spoto views the film as dealing with the attraction towards death, as well as with 'psychic vertigo—the desire to let go, to fall, to float through space, combined with the fear of falling' (Spoto, 1976, p. 308; compare Quinodoz, 1990). He examines Scottie's predicament empathetically: his increasing lack of freedom, his identification with his idealised love object, his panic and subsequent breakdown after he fails to rescue her from (what he is led to perceive as) her fall, and his evolving resemblance of Elster as he attempts to recreate Madeleine. Spoto states: 'Tragically, no one is capable here of reaching the fulfillment of a human involvement—neither Scottie, nor Midge, nor Gavin Elster nor Judy' (p. 303). He suggests that the film exposes 'the ways of false love ... exploitative narcissism on the one hand, and neurotic self-annihilation on the other' (p. 329). His concluding statement is:

The film conveys ... the struggle between the constant yearning for the ideal, and the necessity of living in a world that is far from ideal, whose people are frail and imperfect. It is a film of uncanny maturity and insight, and if its characters are flawed, that is, after all, only a measure of their patent humanity, and of the film's unsentimental yet profound compassion (1976, p. 337).

Wood (1977) shows how the original story of Pierre Boileau and Thomas Narcejac, D'Entre les Morts, with its 'easy pessimism that is as much a sentimental self-indulgence as its opposite' and characters that are 'either helpless devitalised dupes ... or the ingeniously malignant intriguers who trap them' (p. 77), is transformed by Hitchcock into a tragic portrayal 'of the immense value of human relationships and their inherent incapacity of perfect realisation' (p. 78). He analyses the newly added figure of Midge, 'devoid of mystery or reserve', though 'one senses ... a discrepancy between what she is and what she might be' (p. 79), and its contrast to the figure of Madeleine, 'so much more erotic because of its combination of grace, mysteriousness and vulnerability', who 'becomes our dream as well as Scottie's' (p. 82). Wood (1977) traces the way in which, in the second half of the film, our consciousness becomes split between the points of view of Scottie and of Judy, and the pain aroused by Scottie's inability to see the 'real' Judy due to his clinging to 'the ghost of Madeleine that lurks within her' (p. 93). Eventually, Wood suggests, 'Scottie's vertigo is cured ... by finally learning the whole truth' (p. 94), 'yet his cure has destroyed at a blow both the reality and the illusion of Judy/Madeleine, has made the illusion of Madeleine's death real ... Triumph and tragedy are indistinguishibly fused' (p. 95).

Returning to *Vertigo* with added perspective, Wood (1989) analyses the opening of the film (the chase and the policeman's fall) as 'the most extreme and abrupt instance of enforced audience identification in all of Hitchcock' (p. 380), involving the demise of the father/superego, during its failed attempt to control the criminal/id, with the guilty son/ego left hanging (fig. 11). Elster is the new father 'outside the law', the Devil, tempting Scottie by offering him his own wife as wandering Scottie's feminine mirrorimage.

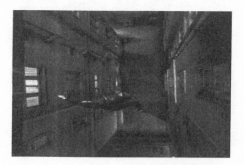

Fig. 11: The policeman's fall

Wood portrays the 'original desire' for mother's breast as an illusion, as the mystifying root of sexuality which must remain mystified;

'"Madeleine" dies (both times) at the moments when she threatens to become a real person' (p. 385).

Wexman's (1986) perspective is Marxist. She criticises Mulvey's psychoanalytic ideas, seeing them as representing 'an idealist position, which ... can obscure the workings of more culturally specific codes within the cinematic text' (p. 36). She discusses the commercialised eroticism of the American film industry, and the way its demands led to controlling Kim Novak's image and to harrassing the actress during production. She unearths 'buried references to issues of class and race' (p. 38) in this film: 'Madeleine's upper-class image entails its opposite: the lower-class Judy' (p. 37); Elster's nostalgia for the days men had 'freedom and power' glorifies exploitative chauvinism and imperialism, whose victims are personified in the Spanish Carlotta Valdes. Wexman concludes that 'Hitchcock has masked the ideological workings of racism and xenophobia beneath a discourse of sexuality which is itself idealized as romantic love' (p. 40).

In another challenge to Mulvey, Keane (1986) contests the view that the camera in *Vertigo* allies itself exclusively with a male point of view. While Mulvey views voyeurism as purely active and sadistic, Keane suggests —with the help of Freud's work on scopophilia—that Scottie also suffers in his voyeuristic position, is acted upon, is in a way a passive character.

The Orphic allusions of *Vertigo* are elaborated by Brown (1986), who notices that in the original novel the hero, Roger Flavieres, repeatedly calls the heroine 'my little Eurydice'. The Orphic story is doubled here, and in both rounds Scottie loses his beloved by 'looking' at her, by pursuing her secret too zealously. Through an analysis of the sequence of scenes, Brown demonstrates how the battles in the film are waged on two vastly different grounds, that of the tragic hero and that of the artist-hero. As a tragic hero, Scottie is guilty of a form of hubris that leads him to reject ordinary, life-affirming love to seek an ideal love that is connected from the outset with 'someone dead'. Put another way, Scottie rejects existential reality in order to live within mythic nonreality (p. 34).

In Brown's analysis, Scottie is also 'the third in a line of men ... who were able to exercise the power of life and death through the sacrifice of three women—Carlotta, Madeleine Elster, and Judy Barton' (p. 37). They are all Apollonian combatants struggling with the female-dominated forces of the Dionysian. In this vein, and in the context of the film's Christian symbolism, Brown interprets the final scene as Scottie's mythic victory over death through the sacrifice of Judy.

Burgin (1986), discussing the film viewer's experience (see Berman, 1998), relates Scottie's urges to the oedipal rescue fantasy towards 'fallen women' analysed by Freud: 'A man rescuing a woman from water in a dream means that he makes her ... his own mother' (Freud, 1910, p. 174).

Goodkin (1987) relates the story of *Vertigo* to central themes in Proust, including the centrality of a 'Madeleine' (the cake, in Proust's case) as an embodiment of a central experience of reliving the past; both works portray controlling and freezing the passage of time by turning life into art. In both, he suggests, the world of men is singularly unkind to the protagonists, who crave maternal support (fig. 12 opposite).

Palombo (1987), on the other hand, interprets Scottie's fainting in Midge's apartment as revealing his 'raging fear of his dependence on Midge and her mothering ... Mother's bosom has been revealed as both the parapet to which Ferguson clings for dear life ... and as the abyss into which he must fall when the crack-up comes' (p. 49). He describes Scottie's quest to decipher Madeleine's dream as parallel to a similar search in Hitchcock's earlier Spellbound, but this time the results are demoralising to the viewer; while frustrating our wish for a straightforward solution, they allow—Palombo suggests —'a much deeper investigation of the dream substrate of waking life' (p. 52). Scottie's subsequent nightmare 'shows how closely Madeleine's dream fits Ferguson's inner emotional state' (p. 53), and first expresses the possibility that he is Elster's victim.

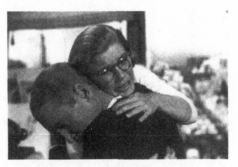

Fig. 12: Scottie faints in Midge's arms

Palombo notices how the viewer's identification with Scottie is disturbed by the flashback scene; from that point on we watch his struggle 'from the viewpoint of a parent, perhaps, but no longer from that of another self' (p. 55). Contrary to many of his other films, here 'Hitchcock declined the role of benevolent overseer, leaving Ferguson and Judy to fight the demoralizing effects of Elster's plot with their own limited emotional resources' (p. 61).

While Palombo discusses Scottie as dream interpreter, Rothman (1987) appears to be the first to speak of 'his role as investigator, but also as therapist' (p. 66). His project in the first part of the film 'becomes a calling ... on which he stakes his entire being. By explaining everything, he ... will save and win this damsel in distress'. In analysing the second part Rothman emphasises that 'no matter how violently Scottie treats Judy ... his goal is to liberate this woman's self, not suppress it. Further-more, he is acting out of love for this woman ... [who] wishes for Scottie to bring Madeleine back' (pp. 71-2). Rothman does not believe Hitchcock indicts Scottie's project: 'what gives rise to Scottie's monstrousness is his heroic refusal to let his love be lost and his equally heroic willingness to plunge into the unknown. His failure is a tragedy' (p. 72).

Rothman's view of Judy as 'unfinished, uncreated' (1987, p. 71) and therefore longing to be allowed to develop into 'Madeleine', is echoed in Poznar's interpretation: 'Scottie knows Judy can become Madeleine, that what is most beautiful in her can only be realised if she has the courage to accept the potential Madeleine in her' (1989, p. 59). Poznar's admiration of Scottie and Madeleine makes him judge some figures— and some scholars—severely: '[Midge] is as imperceptive and unfeel-ing as Elster ... And no less imperceptive and brutal are the comments of the coroner who utters the kind of judgment on Scottie found in some critics who are as convinced as the coroner that Scottie is the victim of an abnormal and dangerous weakness' (p. 60). 'To renounce the Madeleine in us is to renounce our deepest self', Poznan states (p. 61).

Hollinger (1987) points out that the film works through a female oedipal drama, and the desire it portrays for unity with a powerful maternal presence (Carlotta) subverts its masculine premises. She views Scottie as striving to break off his relationship with the maternal.

Modleski (1988) returns to the question of the film's supposed male viewpoint, and suggests that 'the male spectator is as much "deconstructed" as constructed' by Hitchcock, due to his 'fascination with femininity which throws masculine identity into question and crisis' (p. 87). Scottie's 'desire to merge with a woman who in some sense doesn't exist ... points to self-annihilation' (p. 94). At the same time, his 'very effort to cure her, which is an effort to get her to mirror man and his desire, to see [his] reason, destroys woman's otherness' (p. 95). In his nightmare, 'Scottie actually lives out Madeleine's hallucination ... and he dies Madeleine's death. His attempts at a cure having failed, he himself is plunged into the "feminine" world of psychic disintegration, madness, and death' (p. 95). Modleski concludes that the film solicits 'a masculine bisexual identification because of the way the male character oscillates between ... a hypnotic and masochistic fascination with the woman's desire and a sadistic attempt to gain control over her' (p. 99)—fig. 13 below: Scottie's nightmare:

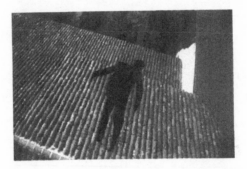

Brill (1988) focuses on 'the failure of Scottie to discover himself in love', in contrast to Hitchcock's romantic films in which quests lead 'to the creation (or recovery) through love of the protagonists' personal and social identities' (p. 207). 'No greater horror can occur in a Hitchcock movie than the failure or exploitation of the instinct to love and heal, on which the recovery of innocence ultimately depends' (p. 211). He points to the anti-redemptive meaning of the Christian images in the film, and to its ironic 'tendency toward self-deconstruction ... the incorporation in every proposition of its contrary' (p. 214). 'The desire to possess one's lover is closely bound ... to a passion for knowing, for formulating and fixing reality ... [but] Scottie and Judy need love, not knowledge' (p. 218).

White (1991) summarises many authors who view *Vertigo* as dealing with the impossible position into which the woman is placed, with her unknownness and her eerie knowledge; as arousing sympathy for her plight. 'Judy, like Scottie, may be looking for a replacement for a lost loved one, in this case her father' (p. 915); Scottie risks death, but it is the woman, 'his more vulnerable other, the part of him that is umbilically tied to the mother, who dies' (p. 919). White, however, calls for an allegorical reading of the film, emphasising 'the non-self, the divided self, what de Man, after Baudelaire, calls the ironic self' (p. 931). Challenging certain feminist idealisations, she points out that 'the desire to merge with the mother is ... extraordinarily threatening to the daughter, too' (p. 926).

Cohen (1995) describes *Vertigo* as transitional in Hitchcock's abandonment of the legacy of Victorian culture, and particularly of the Victorian notions of character and of gender complementarity, moving towards his later 'character effacing' films. Cohen compares the Carlotta story to novels of George Eliot or Thomas Hardy, and describes the film's reversals (constant 'spiraling back upon itself') as 'a deconstructive insight ... into the way nineteenth-century male novelists can be said to have constructed female subjectivity and then passed it on to film-makers like Hitchcock as the real thing' (p. 139).

After realising Madeleine was 'constructed' we want Scottie to love the 'real' Judy, which in many ways is no less a construction. Cohen expresses 'a postmodern recognition ... that experience is, by definition, constructed and hence delusionary' (p. 141).

Gabbard's (1998) analysis of the film emphasises the defensive side in the objectification of women, often involved in men's sexuality. He underlines 'the need for omnipotent, and even sadistic, control of the love object to deal with the terror of object loss at the core of male desire'. Contempt, he suggests, lies underneath the surface of Scottie's symbiotic needs and idealisation of women. Gabbard relates this theme to Hitchcock's own 'lifelong struggles with dependency, women and sadism', documented by several biographical episodes.

Quinodoz (personal communication, 1996) applies to the film her object-relations interpretation of clinical vertigo (Quinodoz, 1990), seen as a warning system preventing the patient from being overwhelmed by his or her split-off infantile part. In the first part of the film, she suggests, the spectator—like Scottie—is overwhelmed by contradictory information: 'What is real? Are the events happening to Madeleine real? Magic? Madness? Are they fantasies? Lies? A plot?' In the last scene, Scottie overcomes his vertigo when he is sure of being in a realistic world, while Judy—who was throughout the film reality-oriented, and free of vertigo—is overwhelmed by the magic world, and by sudden (and lethal) vertigo, when she sees the nun.

AN OVERVIEW

Our reading of *The Turn of the Screw* would thus attempt not so much to capture the mystery's solution, but to follow, rather, the significant path of its flight; not so much to solve or answer the enigmatic question of the text, but to investigate its structure; not so much to name and make explicit the ambiguity of the text, but to understand the necessity and the rhetorical functioning of the textual ambiguity (Felman, 1982, p. 119).

Comparing the divergent interpretations offered of *Vertigo* is intriguing (see Werman, 1979). We may notice contradictions related to changes in zeitgeist. Mulvey's militant feminism, in which males are mostly exploiters, contrasts with the subtler feminism of Modleski or White, in which men and women alike are damaged by rigid role-models. Similarly, earlier interpretations taking the plot at facevalue, differ from Cohen's post-modernist scepticism, highlighting the film's deconstruction of its own narrative. Other contrasts can be traced to the way theory is utilised: Mulvey mobilises Freud's work on perversions for her ideological purposes, missing its subtleties, while Keane reads Freud much more carefully, enriching our understanding of the film's nuances. On an additional level, many variations in the way *Vertigo* is seen can be related to (counter)transference reactions of the writers to the film, to its protagonists, and to its creator.

My use of the atypical term (counter)transference conveys my view that the deeper experiences of analyst and analysand are not inherently different, in spite of their distinct roles and goals in the analytic encounter; distinguishing transference from countertransference may be superficial. This view originates in a long tradition within psychoanalysis, starting with Ferenczi (Berman, 1996) and culminating in the recent contributions of Ogden, Mitchell and many other authors, who conceptualise the analytic situation as inherently relational or intersubjective (Berman, 1997). This development accounts for the growing realisation within clinical psychoanalysis that the patient's transference often involves genuine attempts to interpret the analyst's personality (Aron, 1991; Gill, 1982), while the analyst's interpretive work is often coloured—and potentially inspired —by countertransference (Racker, 1968; Renik, 1993).

This new frame of reference has given valuable inspiration to the psychoanalytic exploration of literature and art (Berman, 1991, 1993a). The reader's, viewer's and listener's experience, whether they are laymen or professional critics and scholars, can also be conceived as combining an attempt to uncover and spell out the work's meanings with unavoidably personal emotional reactions and identifications. The return of subjectivity (and then intersubjectivity) into psychoanalysis coincides with recent trends in literary and art scholarship, such as readerresponse criticism and deconstruction, both moving away from assuming 'objective' meanings as fixed properties of works of art.

The question of *Vertigo*'s 'real' meaning becomes pointless, if we assume that the film acquires a unique meaning for each viewer, influenced by her or his inner world. In other words, we are now talking neither of a hidden true content that can be objectively deciphered (an assumption inherent in classical versions of 'applied analysis'), nor of interpretation as 'merely a projection' of the viewer, but rather of a new individual significance emerging in the unique transitional space opened up by the viewer's encounter with the emotional universe of the film.

While in literature we may speak of an intersubjective exchange between author and reader, mediated by the text and by the transitional space created by reading, in arts such as theatre and film the process is more complex. 'Written drama, on its way to the viewer, meets several readers—director, actors, designers, musicians—each of whom develops out of his or her inner world an interpretive understanding of the play' (Berman, 1991, p. 8). In a parallel way, we could explore the way Hitchcock reacted to the original story and transformed it (Spoto, 1983; Wood, 1977), or attempt to study the impact on the film of his complex interaction with actors James Stewart and Kim Novak, hoping to transcend the one-sided (counter)transferential focus of Wexman (and Gabbard) on Novak as Hitchcock's victim.

My choice to write in this context of (counter)transference also hints at an inherent conflict between two potential reactions, neither of which should be taken for granted. The reader's or spectator's response may be experienced mostly as an analyst's countertransference, when figures, work of art or artist are primarily viewed as enigmatic, as needing to be explained, and at the extreme end as being pathological. Alternately, the reader's or spectator's emotional set may be closer to an analysand's transference, when the work, its protagonists or its creator are primarily experienced as valuable and a source of insight. These different starting points usually lead towards opposing views—see fig. 14 below: Midge and the mock portrait.

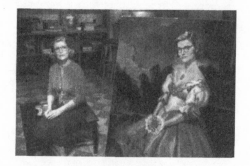

(Counter)transference is only rarely spelled out by critics (Cohen describes her 'wave of irritation that that necklace gave it all away'; 1995, pp. 140-41), but it is omnipresent. Its role can be detected, for example, in the divergent ways in which Midge is portrayed by various authors. When Midge paints her own face into Carlotta Valdez's portrait, this is seen as a brave demystificatory act by Modleski (1988, p. 90) and as 'a travesty, a degradation ... a profound blasphemy' by Poznar (1989, p. 61), who deeply identifies with Scottie's romantic vision. Gabbard (1998) emphasises Midge's maternal qualities, the soothing tone of her voice, while Cohen speaks of her as 'a male imitation ... who presents herself as Scottie's buddy and whose rule of life seems to be to keep a stiff upper lip' (1995, p. 139). Hollinger (1987) describes Midge as a spectator figure, with whom the female spectator identifies uneasily, while White (1991, p. 926) emphasises her actual ignorance of Scottie's situation.

(Counter)transference also colours the way Scottie and Judy/Madeleine are portrayed by the critics, in ways too numerous to be listed. In her brilliant meta-analysis of the critical readings of The Turn of the Screw, Felman (1982) demonstrates how the debate around the story recreates many of its basic emotional themes. Similarly, the rescue fantasy, a central motive in *Vertigo*, is recreated when various scholars strive to rescue Judy from Scottie, rescue both from Elster (who appears to be forgotten in analyses emphasising Scottie's pathology) or from constrictive gender roles, rescue Judy from 'Madeleine' or vice versa, rescue Scottie from the coroner's wrath and from other scholars, or rescue Kim Novak from Hitchcock. (The latter instance is particularly revealing, as one wonders: what will Beauty/Novak do when rescued from Beast/Hitchcock—go back into playing Miss Deepfreeze in commercials, as Novak did shortly before creating, in collaboration with Hitchcock, this role of a lifetime?)

My own basic interpretation, outlined earlier on, was initially formulated and presented after viewing the film and reading only Spoto (1976) and Wood (1977). It undoubtedly expresses my own (counter)transference, as evidenced by my lifelong preoccupation with the impact of rescue fantasies (e.g. Berman, 1988, 1993b) and their role in our work.

While Freud first spoke of rescue fantasies in 1910, it was Ferenczi who described a parallel phenomenon in analysis, when 'the doctor has unconsciously made himself his patient's patron or knight' (Ferenczi, 1919, p. 188). Only half a century later the term rescue fantasy was directly applied to analysts, by Greenacre (1966, p. 760). Contrary to Freud's oedipal focus (an underlying wish to rescue mother from father), my own interpretation of the rescue fantasy, spelled out in the first section of the paper, emphasises the object of rescue as a projected version of the rescuer's own disavowed vulnerability, and the danger from which rescue is needed—as a split-off version of the rescuer's aggression. The resultant interaction I describe can be compared to a mutual transference-countertransference enactment, of the kind that can be used therapeutically if brought to consciousness and understood (Renik, 1993), but may also be destructive when it remains unconscious, when its significance is denied or rationalised away.

Reading the rest of the literature on *Vertigo* more recently gave me a sense of validation, enabled me to refine several formulations, and made me aware of problematic aspects of others. One of the latter was my initial confidence that 'real Judy' resents the role of 'Madeleine', and agrees to assume it anew only as a way to find Scottie's love. My contemplation of the paradoxical nature of 'seeming' and 'being' for the protagonists of Graham Greene (Berman, 1995), helped me realise that for Hitchcock in this film, as for Greene in *The Comedians*, the nature of the subject is enigmatic and far from firm certainty. I found Cohen's comment about the viewer's yearning to find an authentic self (1995, p. 139) a good description of my initial experience.

Cohen's (1995) analysis of the major difference between the firm 'Victorian' identity of L. B. Jeffries in *Rear Window* and the shaky identity of Scottie (both played by Stewart) points to the risk in equating the two figures—and the two films—due to similarities of content (voyeurism, rescue, disability) —see fig. 15 below: Scottie in the final scene.

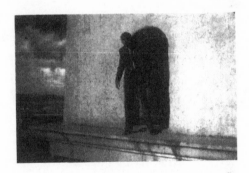

Such contents can be easily tied to Hitchcock's own pathology, as suggested by Almansi (1992), in the tradition of psychoanalytic pathography, which is characterised by an unacknowledged global (counter)transference: artist and figures are seen as sick patients. While Gabbard's (1998) emphasis on object loss (a view congruent

with my own) radically differs from Mulvey's (1975) emphasis on castration anxiety, they are both influenced by this pathographic tradition. Spitz comments: 'Pathography ... assumes that creative activity
does not represent for the artist a real "working through" of basic conflict ... This view severely limits the pathographer's capacity to deal
with aspects of creating that are relatively conflict-free ... [and] fails
to deal with those aspects of the artist's intention that arise in response
to the reality of the developing work itself' (1985, pp. 51-2).

In addition, I would argue, pathography alienates us from works of
art studied, allows a defensive distancing in which work and artist alike
are 'not us'. (Hitchcock or his envoy Scottie have voyeuristic needs; we
don't.) Therefore, it blinds us to the ways we could—as psychoanalysts—truly learn from art, rather than offer it our preconceived
understanding. Of course, creative and unconventional art has a better
potential to 'become our analyst' rather than 'our disturbed patient'.
(When using these codes we should not forget how often we 'learn
from the patient', so that roles are reversed in the clinical situation as
well.) The comparison of *Spellbound* and *Vertigo* is useful here.

Spellbound (1945), while excellently crafted, is a deeply conventional film. We cannot learn much from it, because it learned too
dutifully from us—namely, it offers a simplified version of an analytic cure through effective dream interpretation, all 'by the book'
(those books popular in the US in the nineteen forties, in which
psychoanalysis was glorified as a cure-all). The destructive potential of the therapeutic encounter is split off into the demonic (male)
figure of 'the mad doctor', which leaves the idealised version of the
(female) analyst-rescuer-lover pure, effective (with the help of an
omniscient father-figure) and victorious. It's great entertainment,

but a far cry from the complex emotional realities of actual analytic practice.

Vertigo (1958) is in some ways its negative. It represents Hitchcock's artistic maturation, a freedom to cast doubt upon conventional wisdoms, including the power of psychoanalytic interpretation as a method of establishing objective reality, as well as a vehicle of rescue. Like its predecessor, interpretation plays a major role, but—as I portrayed in the first part of this paper—a role that is illusory. In deconstructing our rescue myth, Hitchcock gets closer to the subtle emotional paradoxes and dilemmas that haunt all helping professions. 'Hitchcock's apparent loss of faith in the psychological power of the truth revealed in dreams' actually allows him 'a much deeper investigation of the dream substrate of waking life' (Palombo, 1987, p. 52)—see fig. 16 below: Hitchcock in *Vertigo.*

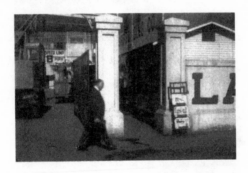

Interpretation, of course, was not invented by Freud. In an intriguing study comparing change processes in psychoanalysis and in drama, Simon offers the following definition: 'Tragedy is that art form which, by means of representation of significant human actions

... progressively analyzes and, by means of continuous interpretation of those actions, painfully lays bare their range of meanings and implications ... The inexorable and irreversible aspects of the tragedy are the correlates of the process of continuous misinterpretation' (1985, p. 399).

Simon gives several examples in which inexact and unempathetic interpretations (e.g. by the chorus in *Antigone*, by the Fool in *King Lear*) push the protagonists towards disaster. Indeed, Midge's interpretation of Scottie's love for Madeleine can be seen as exactly this kind of inexact unempathetic interpretation, which alienates Scottie from Midge and makes him utterly lonely; while Scottie's illusory omniscient interpretation of Madeleine's dream plays a role in the process culminating in Judy's death.

Related questions are raised by Jacobson (1989) in his re-evaluation of Freud's and Jones's views of *Hamlet*. While casting doubt on the search for the play's hidden *a priori* 'meaning', Jacobson points out the preoccupation of the play with the problems and pitfalls inherent in the mutual interpretations offered by its protagonists to each other: 'All the men and women in it do their best to understand the actions of those with whom they are involved, as they have to. But what they most effectively reveal to us in their attempts is—themselves ... It is because we know our understanding to be so partial that we are bound to attend as closely as we can to whatever is before us; and in so doing to attend also to the terms in which we try to comprehend it ... This ... is true not only for the characters in the play, but also for each of its readers ...' (1989, pp. 270-1).

So, while we will never reach a definitive interpretation of *Vertigo*'s meaning, this fascinating film can help us interpret ourselves, and develop a finer understanding of our relations as psychoanalysts with art, with our clinical work, and with ourselves.

REFERENCES

ALMANSI, R. J. (1992). Alfred Hitchcock's disappearing women: a study in scopophilia and object loss. *Int. J. Psychoanal.*, 19: 81-90.

ARON, L. (1991). Symposium on 'Reality and the analytic relationship': the patient's experience of the analyst's subjectivity. *Psychoanal. Dialogues*, 1: 29-51.

BERMAN, E. (1988). Communal upbringing in the Kibbutz: the allure and risks of psychoanalytic utopianism. *Psychoanal. Study Child*, 43: 319- 335.

—— (1991). Psychoanalysis and theater: imaginary twins? *Assaph: Studies in the Theater*, 7: 1-19.

—— (1993a). Introduction to *Essential Papers on Literature and Psychoanalysis*, ed. E. Berman. New York: New York Univ. Press.

—— (1993b). Psychoanalysis, rescue and utopia. *Utopian Studies*, 4:44- 56.

—— (1995). Review of R. Pierloot, Psychoanalytic Patterns in the Work of Graham Greene. *Int. J. Psychoanal.*, 76: 865-867.

—— (1996). The Ferenczi renaissance. *Psychoanal. Dialogues*, 6:391- 411.

—— (1997). Relational psychoanalysis: a historical background. *Amer. J. Psychother.*, 51: 185-203.

—— (1998). The film viewer: from dreamer to dream interpreter. *Psychoanal. Inq.*, 18: 193-206.

BRILL, L. (1988). *The Hitchcock Romance: Love and Irony in Hitchcock's Films.* Princeton, NJ: Princeton Univ. Press.

BROWN, R. S. (1986). *Vertigo* as orphic tragedy. *Literature Film Q.,* 14:32-43.

BURGIN, V. (1986). Diderot, Barthes, *Vertigo.* In *Formations of Fantasy,* ed. V. Burgen et al. London: Methuen, pp. 85-108.

COHEN, P. M. (1995). *Alfred Hitchcock: The Legacy of Victorianism.* Lexington: Univ. Press Kentucky.

DONNE, J. (1624). Devotions. In *Selections from Divine Poems, Sermons, Devotions and Prayers,* ed. J. Booty. New York: Paulist Press, 1990.

FELMAN, S. (1982). Turning the screw of interpretation. In *Literature and Psychoanalysis.* Baltimore, MD: Johns Hopkins Univ. Press, pp. 94-207.

FERENCZI, S. (1919). On the technique of psychoanalysis. In *Further Contributions to the Theory and Technique of Psycho-Analysis.* New York: Brunner-Mazel, 1980, pp. 177-189.

FREUD, S. (1910). A special type of object choice made by men. *S.E.* 11.

GABBARD, G. O. (1998). *Vertigo:* female objectification, male desire, and object loss. *Psychoanal. Inq.,* 18: 161–7.

GILL, M. M. (1982). *Analysis of Transference.* New York: Int. Univ. Press.

GOODKIN, R. E. (1987). Film and fiction: Hitchcock's *Vertigo* and Proust's 'vertigo'. *Mod. Lang. Notes,* 102: 1171-1181.

GREENACRE, P. (1966). *Emotional Growth.* New York: Int. Univ. Press.

HOLLINGER, K. (1987). The look, narrativity, and the female spectator in *Vertigo. J. Film & Video,* 39:18-27.

JACOBSON, D. (1989). Hamlet's other selves. *Int. J. Psychoanal.,* 16: 265-272.

KAPLAN, E. N. (ED.) (1990). *Psychoanalysis and Cinema.* New York & London: Routledge.

KEANE, M. (1986). A closer look at scopophilia: Mulvey, Hitchcock, and *Vertigo.* In *A Hitchcock Reader,* ed. M. Deutelbaum & L. Poague. Ames, IA: Iowa State Univ. Press, pp. 231-248.

MODLESKI, T. (1988). *The Women who Knew Too Much: Hitchcock and Feminist Theory.* London: Methuen.

MULVEY, L. (1975). *Feminism and Film Theory,* ed. C. Penley. New York: Routledge, 1988, pp. 570. Visual pleasure and narrative cinema. *Screen,* 16: 6-18. Reprinted in *Feminism and Film Theory,* ed. C. Penley. New York: Routledge, 1988, pp. 57-68.

PALOMBO, S. R. (1987). Hitchcock's *Vertigo:* the dream function in film. In *Images in Our Souls: Cavell, Psychoanalysis, and Cinema,* ed. J. H. Smith & W. Kerrigan. Baltimore: Johns Hopkins Univ. Press, pp. 44-63.

POZNAR, W. (1989). Orpheus descending: love in *Vertigo. Literature Film Q.,* 17:59-65.

QUINODOZ, D. (1990). Vertigo and object relationship. *Int. J. Psychoanal.,* 71: 53-63.

RACKER, H. (1968). *Transference and Countertransference.* London: Karnac, 1982.

RENIK, O. (1993). Countertransference enactment and the psychoanalytic process. In *Psychic Structure and Psychic Change,* ed. M. Horowitz et al. Madison, CT: Int. Univ. Press, pp. 135-158.

ROTHMAN, W. (1987). *Vertigo:* the unknown woman in Hitchcock. In *Images in Our Souls: Cavell, Psychoanalysis, and Cinema,* ed. J. H. Smith & W. Kerrigan. Baltimore: Johns Hopkins Univ. Press, pp. 64-81.

SIMON, B. (1985). 'With cunning delays and evermounting excitement': or, what thickens the plot in psychoanalysis and tragedy? In *Psychoanalysis: The Vital Issues, Vol. II*, ed. J. Gedo & G. Pollock. New York: Int. Univ. Press, pp. 387-435.

SPITZ, E. H. (1985). *Art and Psyche: A Study in Psychoanalysis and Aesthetics* New Haven, CT: Yale Univ. Press.

SPOTO, D. (1976). *The Art of Alfred Hitchcock*. New York: Hopkinson & Blake. (Revised edition: Doubleday, 1992.)

—— (1983). *The Dark Side of Genius: The Life of Alfred Hitchcock*. New York: Ballentine.

WERMAN, D. (1979). Methodological problems in the psychoanalytic interpretation of literature: a review of studies on Sophocles' *Antigone. J. Amer. Psychoanal. Assn.*, 27: 451-478.

WEXMAN, V. W. (1986). The critic as consumer: film study at the university, *Vertigo*, and the film canon. *Film Q*, 39:32-41.

WHITE, S. (1991). Allegory and referentiality: *Vertigo* and feminist criticism. *Mod. Lang. Notes*, 106: 910-932.

WOOD, R. (1977). *Hitchcock's Films*. South Brunswick: Barnes.

—— (1989). *Hitchcock's Films Revisited*. New York: Columbia Univ. Press.

4. NEIL JORDAN'S *THE CRYING GAME*

GLEN O. GABBARD, TOPEKA, KS

In Neil Jordan's 1992 film *The Crying Game*, a British soldier named Jody (Forest Whitaker) is taken hostage by a group of Irish terrorists. In the course of his brief captivity, he develops a friendship with one of his captors named Fergus (Stephen Rea). Realising that he may never emerge from his ordeal alive, Jody shows a picture of his girlfriend Dil to Fergus and tells him to look her up when the dust settles if anything happens to him. After Jody is killed in a freak accident, Fergus heads to London and locates Dil, only to fall in love with her. To his great horror and to the audience's considerable surprise, Dil turns out to be a cross-dressing male.

The Crying Game was the film industry's sleeper hit in 1992, making about $62 million at the box office. The success of the movie was largely related to the way it was marketed—namely, a film with a secret that nobody, not even the critics, was revealing. This shrewd strategy drew people because they thought they were going to see a thriller rather than a love story with strong homosexual themes. Once the audience took their seats in the darkened theatre, they watched a narrative unfold that repeatedly set up situations only to knock them down. In the opening scene, ironically accompanied by a blaring rendition of 'When a Man Loves a Woman', Jody tries to pick up a woman at a carnival. The audience assumes that Jody is a straight male. The first jolt is delivered when they discover that the woman he has picked up is a terrorist who has laid a trap for him.

The next twist is that one terrorist is nothing like a terrorist at all. Instead, the audience enjoys the development of a poignantly close relationship between Jody and Fergus, one that is homo-erotically tinged by a scene in which Fergus must hold the penis of Jody (whose hands are tied) so he can urinate. While the major surprise is the discovery that Dil (Jaye Davidson) is actually a male, a more profound and unexpected development is that Fergus continues to love Dil even after this jarring revelation.

Why did the secret of Dil's genital configuration become so over-valued among viewers of the film? The artifice of a man dressed as a woman, of course, is not new. Cross-dressing for purposes of disguise was a convention of Elizabethan comedy. Shakespeare exploited it for his purposes. What both Neil Jordan and Shakespeare suggest is that the heterosexual norm is a highly unstable state regularly subject to infiltrations from homo-erotic desires.

Stoller (1975) pointed out that dividing people into homosexuals and heterosexuals is highly problematic. He stressed that heterosexuality is no more natural or normal than homosexuality and that we would do better to speak of 'the homosexualities' and 'the heterosexualities'. Jordan's film reminds us that we are all on shaky ground when it comes to our sexual identities and preferences. As every analyst steeped in the transference–countertransference configurations of an ongoing analysis knows, these are fluid and subject to influences from the unconscious that we may consciously find unacceptable (Gabbard & Wilkinson, 1996).

The Crying Game can also be understood as providing the audience with the opportunity to revisit and master a universal developmental crisis involving curiosity about the genitalia of the opposite sex. Children in the pre-oedipal phase often believe with conviction that they can have all qualities of both genders (Fast, 1984). Observations of children (Roiphe & Galenson, 1981) suggest that awareness of anatomical gender difference occurs in both boys and girls during the rapprochement sub-phase of separation-individuation. This recognition signals a period of mourning that accompanies the realisation that gender entails limits. For the boy child, it may also trigger anxiety that his genitals may be vulnerable. Stoller suggested that when a man dresses as a woman, he concretises the unconscious fantasy that a woman really does have a penis (i.e. she is not castrated). Yet the fantasy of the phallic woman (or mother) is not simply reassuring to the boy child— it also resonates with a darker concern that an omnipotent, penetrating mother may take advantage of his vulnerability (Gabbard & Gabbard, 1993).

Hence the revelation in *The Crying Game* taps into this developmental moment with all its associated conflict and ambivalence. Many films have been created around this theme, among them *Tootsie, Some Like It Hot, M. Butterfly, Victor/Victoria*, and *Priscilla, Queen of the Desert*. The usual situation involves a set-up in which the audience knows more than the characters in the film about the true nature of the disguised character's genitals. Of course, we all take smug delight in the discovery of the secret by other characters in the film. An unforgettable moment in Tootsie occurs when Dustin Hoffman takes off his wig and the camera cuts from one reaction shot to another as everyone recoils in horror. The audience members master their own traumatic childhood awakening to genital difference by laughing uproariously at the shock of all the uninformed movie characters.

In *The Crying Game* this artifice is modified so that neither the members of the audience nor the protagonist in the film are aware of Dil's maleness. The spectators share the surprise with Fergus. One unedited shot beginning at Dil's head and ending at his genital region ends with Fergus going into the bathroom to vomit. He is disgusted not only by the image of a phallic woman but also by his own homo-erotic desire. Some audience members have similarly disturbing reactions. After viewing this film with an analytic society, I asked for the audience to share their reactions. One analyst said that he did not see any male genitals at the end of the shot. Another said that he was certain that another actor had been edited into the shot between the head and the crotch. They had seen but not seen the troubling image on the screen, which undoubtedly resonated with earlier experiences of disbelief and shock at the exposure to female genitalia or feelings of desire for another man.

In addition to this re-creation of the dawning awareness of genital difference, Jordan has another, more subversive, agenda. His overarching point is that genitalia do not really matter in the way that we think they do. Neither do racial differences count. Jody and Dil are both black, while Fergus is white. In an early scene in which Jody shows Fergus Dil's picture, he says that she is probably not Fergus's type. The audience is led to think that he is referring to her race. In effect, Jordan refuses to make gender, sexual orientation, race or even politics into 'either/or' issues. The director has been quoted as saying he wanted to make 'a portrait of a guy who, at every stage of the examination of his emotions, thinks he's got the explanation, and at each turn finds out "that's not what I thought I was fascinated with, that's not what it's about, that's not what my relationship with this woman or this man is actually about". In the end he's just left with the bare facts of his own existence and this other person he thought was a woman who's turned out to be a man, but he still likes her' (Taubin, 1993, p. 54).

The point of *The Crying Game*, in my reading of the film, is that we exaggerate the differences between ourselves and others by focusing on the genitals, the choice of love objects, political affiliations, or one's race or culture, while missing the fundamental human capacity to transcend these differences through love. In Jordan's own words, the crucial dividing line is not one of race or sexual orientation; it is 'between the vicious and the generous' (Taubin, 1993, p. 54). In 1918 Freud reflected on Crawley's ideas about the taboo of personal isolation that separates individuals from one another: 'It is precisely the minor differences in people who are otherwise alike that form the basis of feelings of strangeness and hostility between them. It would be tempting to pursue this idea and to derive from this 'narcissism of minor differences' the hostility which in every human relation we see fighting successfully against feelings of fellowship and overpowering the commandment that all men should love one another' (p. 199).

This statement would have served as a fitting coda to *The Crying Game*.

REFERENCES

FAST, I. (1984). *Gender Identity: A Differentiation Model (Advances in Psychoanalysis: Theory, Research, and Practice, Vol. 2)*. Hillsdale, NJ: Analytic Press.

FREUD, S. (1918). The taboo of virginity (Contributions to the psychology of love III.) *S.E.* 11.

GABBARD, K. & GABBARD, G. O. (1993). Phallic women in the contemporary cinema. *Amer. Imago*, 50: 421-439.

GABBARD, G. O. & WILKINSON, S. M. (1996). Nominal gender and gender fluidity in the psychoanalytic situation. *Gender & Psychoanal.*, 1: 463-481.

ROIPHE, H. & GALENSON, E. (1981). *Infantile Origins of Sexual Identity.* New York: Int. Univ. Press.

STOLLER, R. J. (1975). *Perversion: The Erotic Form of Hatred.* New York: Pantheon.

TAUBIN, A. (1993). Mystery man. *The Village Voice*, 19 January, pp. 52-54.

5. HIDDEN IN THE IMAGERY: AN UNCONSCIOUS SCENE IN *THE CONFORMIST*

HERBERT H. STEIN, New York

Bernardo Bertolucci's 1970 film, *The Conformist*, is based on Alberto Moravia's novel about a young man, Marcello, in pre-war Italy, who volunteers his services to the Fascists, not out of ideology, but to blend in, disguising his perverse sado-masochistic tendencies by expressing them through a perverse cultural norm. Bertolucci has changed the focus of Moravia's plot by presenting most of the story through Marcello's reminiscences as he is driven towards the film's central scene, a particularly violent assassination. Marcello has helped set up the assassination of his former teacher, Luco Quadri, but now he is chasing after Quadri's car with the vague hope of saving Quadri's wife, Anna, who has unexpectedly joined him on the fatal trip. The car and Marcello's memories converge on the assassination, making it the intense focal point of the film.

Marcello's reminiscences are presented with the subtle distortions of subjective memory. Through them we share some of Marcello's own confusion about his motives. We see that he harbours anger towards his psychotic father and drug-addicted mother. We also learn that as a child he was the victim of an attempted seduction at the hands of a young man, Lino, and ended up shooting his seducer, leaving him for dead. He marries a woman he does not love and falls in love with a woman he hardly knows. In its subjectivity and uncertainty the film is similar to an analytic hour. If we approach it that way, we can see that hidden in this tale of an abused and tortured man is another, shorter tale of a child and a primal scene fantasy. It is as if we could reconstruct an early screen memory that adds meaning to the current surface.

One clue to the unconscious in an analytic hour is the presence of repetitions. *The Conformist* can easily be seen to have continual repetitions of primal scene imagery, imagery relating to a child witnessing parental intercourse. Throughout the film, each scene contains some obvious elements of the primal scene while other elements are disguised or missing. As viewers, we never experience the primal scene directly, but are continually teased with fragmented primal scene imagery.

For instance, as the film opens Marcello receives a phone call in bed. He prepares to leave, taking a pistol, and covers his sleeping wife's exposed back and buttocks. Here we have important static visual elements of the primal scene—a man and woman in bed, the woman's exposed body, and the symbolic suggestion of the phallus. A few scenes later, Marcello parts a curtain in a government office to see a man beginning to make love over a desktop to a sexually provocative woman. Now, the bed is disguised as a desktop and the nakedness as sexually provocative clothing while the sexual act and the voyeurism are explicit. The child is represented by the adult Marcello, but the visual distortion of this memory sequence makes him look smaller than the figures he is observing. In what will become a pattern, the two scenes contain separated elements of a single image, leaving it to the viewer to bring them together to construct his own preconscious gestalt, blending personal experience and needs with the film's suggestive imagery.

Adjoining scenes add resonance with images of sexual voyeurism. Marcello stares from a darkened radio booth at three attractive singers, describes his sexual embraces with his fiancée, Giulia, to his blind friend, Italo, and has his petting with Giulia interrupted first by her maid and then by her mother. The last of these scenes takes place in Giulia's sitting room, but the light and dark lines of light from the blinds blending with the black and white stripes on Giulia's dress could suggest a view through the slats of a crib.

There are also scenes, scattered throughout the film, that are linked by their repetitive focus on certain visual details. When Marcello peers at the couple through the curtain, the first thing we see is the woman's leg swinging over the side of the desk. In the same scene, the man seems not to see Marcello, but the woman turns to smile back at him. In the course of the film, the camera will focus several times on dangling bare legs and backward stares. There are also reprisals of the opening scene, for example when Marcello, visiting his mother in her bedroom, attempts to cover her partial nakedness and when Lino, the seducer, holding a pistol, undresses while the young Marcello lies on a bed beside him.

In an analytic hour, the repetition of detail can be interpreted as pointing to the presence of an unconscious screen memory (Arlow, 1980). Using a little imagination, we can begin to construct some variation of the following 'screen memory' in *The Conformist*: a child peers up, perhaps through the bars of a crib, as a man undresses and approaches a woman in her bed. The man pulls back the sheet, exposing her nakedness. The child is beckoned and excited by the woman's backward glance at him and her bare leg hanging down.

That hidden 'memory' is further elaborated into a violent fantasy through the assassination and the scene that follows it. The primal scene is not a neutral act. Arlow (1980) has pointed out that it often engenders feelings of envy and desires for revenge from the child who is forced to be a passive observer. Marcello and Quadri capture that envy discussing Plato's parable of the cave in which men are chained to a wall and forced to look at images through a screen. This metaphor applies equally to the passive child forced to view parental sex and the film's audience seated in a theatre, looking up at images on a screen it can never enter. The viewer of *The Conformist*, who is subtly, but repeatedly presented with primal scene imagery, should be primed to identify with that child's excitement and frustration.

As the assassination scene begins, Marcello sits in the rear seat of the car, behind his driver, Mangianello, seemingly paralysed as he watches the events unfold. Quadri and Anna are just ahead of them on a winding mountain road in the midst of a snow-covered forest. Anna looks back over her shoulder (one of the film's repetitive images) at the car following them. She is frightened at being followed, but Quadri is calm and unsuspecting. A car swerves in front of Quadri's car, blocking the way. The driver is slumped over the steering wheel. Anna fears danger and pleads with Quadri not to leave the car. Nevertheless, he goes out to check. Assassins appear from the surrounding woods. The driver of the car steps out to join them. As Quadri asks him what he wants, they begin stabbing him repeatedly. They head for Anna who flees, screaming in terror, as she runs to Marcello's car. Anna presses her face against the rear seat window implicitly begging for him to save her. Marcello does nothing. Anna runs on, the assassins in pursuit. They finally shoot her. She falls to the snow, her face covered with blood.

The scene changes. Several years have passed and Mussolini's government has just been toppled. Marcello says goodnight to his 3- or 4-year-old daughter after leading her in her prayers. He gets a call from his friend, Italo, and prepares to go out to meet him. His wife begs him not to leave (just as Anna had begged Quadri not to leave the car) because there is rioting and danger in the streets in the wake of Mussolini's fall (another assassinated father). Marcello goes out over her objections (as Quadri had). As he leaves, the lights begin to go off and on. The little girl cries out, 'Mommy, where are you? I'm afraid!'

Once again, two scenes can be taken as separate aspects of a single fantasy. The little girl in bed, the parents arguing in the other room, the hint of external danger, and the girl's fright are more mundane elements of the primal scene close to the experience of every viewer. The assassination appears to be far from the bedroom or scenes of childhood, but it conveys the raw emotion and violent imagery that we might associate with the primal scene revenge fantasy. Influenced by the repetitive primal scene imagery that has come before, we can construct the following: a child lies in his bed or crib, perhaps with a nurse nearby (Mangianello), watching his parents in bed, or imagining them together in the next room. He weaves a fantasy of revenge. The parents are interrupted and father leaves, possibly to check on the supposedly sleeping child (the slumped-over driver). This imagery has been suggested in the opening scene when Marcello leaves his bed to go out. The father is viciously murdered and the mother sadistically abused and killed in a more violent version of the primal scene while the child watches, frozen by the scene and his own ambivalence.

Moravia's 1951 novel contains a primal-scene experience with violent overtones that Bertolucci has chosen not to include in the film. Instead, he has, with what I assume to be unconscious artistry, imparted a sense of an unconscious primal scene memory and fantasy that can enrich our experience in a unique way. The success of this unusual dimension will depend upon the ability and need of each viewer preconsciously to reconstruct a scene from its fragmented elements. When it works, it adds depth to the presentation of the film's major political and dynamic themes.

REFERENCES

ARLOW, J. (1980). The revenge motive in the primal scene. *J. Amer. Psychoanal. Assn.*, 28: 519-541.

MORAVIA, A. (1951). *The Conformist.* Trans. A. Davidson. New York: Farrar, Straus and Young.

6. 'AH DOCTOR, IS THERE NOTHIN' I CAN TAKE?': A REVIEW OF *RESERVOIR DOGS*

ADRIENNE HARRIS, NEW YORK

On the surface, Quentin Tarantino's *Reservoir Dogs* (1991) is a grim little crime story about a violently botched jewellery store robbery. It is shot in an odd, discomfiting style that alternates scenes of brutality with comic set pieces filled with wacky male obsessions. The robbery is carried out by a set of losers who have been recruited by an ominous, foul-mouthed father figure who looks, as one of the younger robbers says somewhat admiringly, 'just like The Thing'. A cartoon monster. Although set in the present in Los Angeles, the film and its characters are haunted by the 1970s. Like pentimento, the 1970s are layered through this film, in its soundtrack and aural register and in its visual effect, which is more like that of a low-budget television crime show than a glossy mainstream feature. In its intertextual references to *film noir*, to the conventions of war films and to the popular culture of cartoons, film characters and nineteen-seventies' television as well as its deployment of many signifiers and images, the Vietnam era and the war itself are evoked.

I am going to propose a 'creative misreading' (Bloom, 1973) of this film as an expression of the ungrieved and lingering trauma of Vietnam in American consciousness. Such a reading positions both the film and the spectator in a specific historical and cultural context and is thus precisely not a claim for a universal or generic interpretive approach. In relation to Gabbard's useful taxonomy of methods (1997), I am using here a mixed model drawing on an evolving feminist theory

(Penley, 1989), reception theory, which is a psychoanalytically driven theory of how meaning is evoked and managed (Zizek, 1994) and a psychoanalytic reading of film as the expression of underlying, often unconscious cultural tensions and contradictions. In this film, in particular, a psychoanalytic understanding of trauma and its sequelae may be illuminating.

Vietnam and the American social crisis that followed are never explicitly named, but displaced and buried beneath a modern crime story; the specific horrors of the Vietnam era press on the characters and on the spectator—a trauma that can neither be fully forgotten nor fully remembered. The film disturbs the spectator in many ways. It is structured like a post-traumatic nightmare, the storyline emerging in fragments, in flashbacks, in repetitive returns to scenes of carnage and criminality. Periodically in the film, what we see and what we hear split apart: the screen goes black, the soundtrack continues. The affective mood, often jocular and profane, is set at odds with wrenching violence. The shifting points of view keep the viewer in a disorganised, often dissociated, state.

The war in Vietnam and the cultural time in which it was embedded is carried as an undercurrent most powerfully through the soundtrack. In cars, on the restaurant jukebox, at home and on the road all the characters stay tuned to the same rock programme, a station playing only '70s music. The 'Super Sounds of the 70s', a linking device introduced by the bleak, drugged voice of the disc jockey who triggers the characters' and spectators' haunted memories. Obsessionally he dates the songs he replays (April 1970, May 1974—perhaps uncannily these dates mark the height of the most terrible period of the war). The soundtrack operates paradoxically to soothe and to overstimulate.

While some of the songs are about sedation and drugs (Little Green Bag, Magic Carpet Ride), some are cut directly into scenes of violence. We feel the deeply disjunctive madness in the characters who torture and brutalise against a background of bright, danceable tunes.

The music condenses with another signifier of the war in one of the most disturbing scenes in the film when the psychopathic killer Mr Blond mutilates a policeman he has taken hostage and is interrogating. As he prepares to cut off the man's ear (an iconic or mythic act of castration; a battle trophy enacted upon Vietnamese prisoners and rendered in fictional and non-fictional documentation of that war), he turns on the radio. It is a perverse and unsettling moment. As in so many cinematic images of war and torture, the spectator is voyeuristically implicated, drawn into and stimulated by a horrified tense excess (but still in psychoanalytic terms, a form of pleasure). Suddenly the camera swings away from the scene and we are left to gaze in a dissociated state at the blank brick-wall background, the muffled screams of the cop and the song braided into our aural consciousness.

The link to Vietnam and its difficult social aftermath in America is also made through the film's homage to *film noir*. In the classic *film noir* of the 1940s there is a widely used narrative convention. A man or men wander on to the scene. Sleepwalkers, dazed men, apparently waking from nightmares, they are often amnesiac. They don't know where they belong and in the course of the narrative must be reconnected to family and society. We might see this as the task in all postwar cultures, to bridge the caesura in social life, to reconnect memory, metabolise trauma, fill in the blanks. Shell shock, post-traumatic stress, are ongoing signs of the great ordeal of this task, of its inevitable incompleteness. In *Reservoir Dogs*, men who must forget their names and histories, are convened into a small battalion of criminals. They arrive carrying all the markers of postwar stress: they are melancholy (Mr White), agitated and desperate (Mr Pink), and mad (Mr Blond). The robbery could be seen both as flashback and as retraumatisation. Mr Blond has psychotically shot everyone in the store: a flashback triggered by the alarm. These characters voice the veteran's despair, living in a doomed, embattled, sado-masochistic world in which they can only struggle hopelessly with the uneasy distinctions between friend and foe, loyalty and betrayal, 'professional' and 'psychopath'.

Like Americans' growing turmoil and understanding of the war, the viewer only puts the pieces together slowly. As Mr Pink concludes, 'This thing began as a simple robbery and turned into a bloodbath'. These alienated men exist in a world where bystanders are 'civilians', the most dangerous of whom is a woman. The young undercover cop is shot by such a 'civilian', a woman whose face we never see. This is also a signifier of the war. In several key films about Vietnam (*Full Metal Jacket* and *Platoon* most notably), the most lethal Vietcong enemy was the apparently innocent civilian woman who might nonetheless be secretly armed and deadly.

Yet while these generic tough guys try to practise a macho anonymity and a parody of male military precision and discipline, names and identities keep surfacing. In a trope from the war film genre when personal ties forged through battle and terror connect men, the exchange of names becomes the occasion of tremendous male love and tenderness. In a scene just after a hostage cop has been tortured, the undercover policeman who lies bleeding beside him shoots the psychopathic killer and the two men quietly ask each other's names. We realise that each has protected the identity of the other at enormous cost.

It is always interesting to engage a feminist reading of mainstream film. In this case it is a film that has no women characters and in which masculinity is both comic relief and deadly serious. It was a commonplace of early feminist film criticism, drawing on psychoanalysis, to see the apparatus of cinema as a male form of mastery and to see classical cinema as a seamless organisation and narrative of oedipal drama. In this way cinema is one site in which to observe the constituting of certain subject positions through which sexual difference would be established and maintained. This rather boilerplate version of feminist theory has given way to a greater appreciation of the contradictions and fissures in even the most apparently seamless narratives and to more supple, less monolithic theories of identification. Certainly, *Reservoir Dogs* is a film in which oedipal narratives are parodied or ruptured, and where sexual difference is a source of hysterical anxiety and deadly violence. Far from mastery, male or otherwise, I would read this film as a forced enactment and re-enactment of experience that cannot be mastered.

This film and these characters may be haunted by that other spectre of the nineteen seventies—feminism. Certainly they are preoccupied with women. In the opening scene, the younger men conduct a somewhat hilarious and profane deconstruction of Madonna's song lyrics while the old leader ruminates over his address-book, searching for a woman's lost last name. Finally Mr White shouts: 'I've got Madonna's big dick coming out of my left ear and Toby the Jap coming out of my right' and in one line we have connected male phallic vulnerability (the ear) and the ambiguous position of women, desired but feared. Later Mr White reprises this theme in a melancholy note, remembering his old love, a former partner in crime. 'You push that woman–man thing too long, it gets to you after a while. Hell of a woman. A good little thief.'

Women are powerful and dangerous objects and the fears and fascination they arouse are still best managed with contempt and objectification. Yet in this film the feminine is a position, not an essential identity. Sexual difference is fragile and unreliable yet still an anxious necessity. Throughout the film, the men react to the threat of becoming the degraded Other: woman, black, bitch. Mr Pink doesn't want the name he has been assigned: 'Too faggy'. Mr Blond, newly released from prison, is taunted. 'You've taken so much black semen up your ass that its gone to your brain and out your mouth.' The male body in this film is an endangered object, invaded by blacks and women, shot up and mutilated. Gender panic and sexual panic, interlaced with racist terrors, accelerate through this film, which connects traumatic war memories with the nightmares of an exhausted and demoralised masculinity.

Masculinity is a performance always on the edge of disaster or violence. At the opening credits, the old man leads his gang to the crime, each man dressed identically in dark suits and dark glasses; 'All right, Ramblers, let's get rambling'. The young cop poses in the mirror trying to control his fear. 'You're cool', he tells his image, and conjuring up a TV detective 'Baretta', he leaves his apartment, a barren spot ironically decorated with posters of cartoon heroes. 'An undercover cop is like Marlon Brando', his buddy tells him, a black cop dressed alternately like a hippie or a black revolutionary. In a tough skirmish between two of the robbers, the mad killer suddenly laughs and says, 'You must like Lee Marvin films. Me too'. Old men get the young killed in this film, fathers' authority and the induction of sons into manhood is criminalised and degraded. Masculinity must be made out of the movies.

In a scene that is repeated over the course of the film, the young undercover cop slowly bleeds to death from a gaping stomach wound. Mr White, the loyal wartime buddy, is desperate to save him. To calm the terrified man, he talks to him tenderly, combs his hair and cradles him in his arms. Their eyes are locked in a mutual gaze; this pietà is a moment both homo-erotic and tender. Mother/child, father/son, the gender identities are fluid and ambiguously bisexual. They speak each other's name. 'I'm scared, can't you please hold me.' Mr White comforts Mr Orange with an expertise that sounds born of combat. 'It takes a long time to die. I'm talking days. It takes days to die from your wounds. Time is on your side.' The young cop, a sweetly young male presence in the film, exsanguinates in agony, but this unending painful bleeding, this agonised death that snakes through the film, is also the unstoppable wound of Vietnam.

Names are a powerful signification in this film and this too might be read in relation to the war since the one great national monument to that war is the long Memorial Wall containing the names of the dead. The last scene between two dying men who crawl to a bloody embrace is enigmatic and despairing. Mr White, who has so tenderly combed Mr Orange's hair, holds a gun to the younger man's head. A war in which hatred and destruction raged across class, gender and race lines, at the war and at home, left no one unmaimed or innocent. The song lyrics ironically wail behind the closing credits and the sound of gunshots: 'Doctor. I said Doctor. Is there nothin' I can take to fix this belly ache?'

References

BLOOM, H. (1973). *The Anxiety of Influence: A Theory of Poetry.* London: Oxford Univ. Press.

GABBARD, G. O. (1997). The psychoanalyst at the movies. *Int. J. Psycho-anal.,* 78: 429–434.

PENLEY, C. (1989). *Feminism and Film Theory.* New York: Routledge.

ZIZEK, S. (1994). *The Metastases of Enjoyment.* London: Verso.

7. ARTHUR PENN'S *NIGHT MOVES*: A FILM THAT INTERPRETS US

EMANUEL BERMAN, Israel

'So it's really just a series of concentric circles. The outer reality just goes out and out in those circles; the inner reality, and the inner detective story, is there to be examined—if he would examine it.' Arthur Penn (in Gallagher, 1975, p. 88).

Having been interested in the detective's search as a metaphor for the psychoanalyst's quest, I found myself drawn to *Night Moves* ever since I first saw it. I offer the following interpretive viewing with the assumption that it represents neither an objective deciphering of the film's 'true' meaning, nor solely a projection of my inner world, but rather a new significance that has emerged in the transitional space opened up by my intense personal and transferential encounter with *Night Moves* (Berman, 1997, 1998).

While my earlier thinking focused on the way I could interpret the film, I recently became more cognisant of interpretation as one of the themes in the film itself (as often in drama; Simon, 1985), and of the film *in toto* as an attempted interpretation ('The mystery is inward, and perhaps the solution is inward'; Penn, in Gallagher, 1975, p. 87). Contemporary art has absorbed (sometimes ambivalently) psychoanalytic interpretation, both as a topic and as a tool.

Ellen: 'Who is winning?'
Harry: 'Nobody. One side is losing slower than the other.'

The film's plot interweaves and juxtaposes two equally important stories: detective Harry Mosby's attempt to decipher the disappearance, and later the death, of an adolescent girl, Delly Grastner;
and his struggle to save his disintegrating marriage to Ellen. At the
background of both stories stands a common emotional theme:
failed parenthood, and its sequela—the helpless yearning, despair
and rage of the abandoned child.

Harry (Gene Hackman) was abandoned by his parents as a child,
and brought up by relatives. We hear this story in the context of a
renewed abandonment: his wife's infidelity. Harry discovers the
affair in which Ellen (Susan Clark) is involved, but is unable and
unwilling to speak to her. Instead he violently invades the house of
Marty, Ellen's disabled lover. Marty (Harris Yulin) defends himself
by interpreting: 'I am beginning to get you in focus, Mosby. Ellen
talks a lot about you, how you were left by your parents when you
were very young … It's a clue, isn't that what you do, look for clues?
Didn't you track down your parents? I am sure you were trailing
Ellen when you saw us'.

Marty and Ellen have come to think of Harry's childhood trauma
as the source of his restlessness and action-proneness, of his occupational choice, of his inability to communicate and to invest in family
life (Harry's childlessness at 40 is striking, though never brought
up). Harry is infuriated by Marty's interpretation, but does not dispute it. It eventually appears to enable him to seek renewed closeness with Ellen. In their first intimate conversation, at a later stage,
he finally tells her the truth: he managed with great efforts to find
his father, but upon seeing him on a park bench, 'just a little guy
reading the funny pages out of a paper, mumbling the words

through his lips', he watched for a while and went away, without ever talking to him.

We hear nothing at all about Harry's mother, and wonder: was she dead, or was tracing her more than he could even attempt? Still, a yearning for a motherly bosom appears predominant in the film's visual imagery. The first time we see Harry meeting Ellen he slips his hands into her blouse (but later, right after discovering her affair, he rejects her offer of cocoa); their first open conversation is accompanied by his gently caressing her bare breasts with his toes; another protagonist, Paula (Jennifer Warren), seduces him by telling him of the first time a boy touched her breasts, and by putting his hand on them.

Harry is unexcited, however, when Arlene (Janet Ward), while hiring him to trace her missing daughter, boasts about her own 'lovely tits'. The film makes a sharp distinction between desirable good breasts that can be easily lost (Ellen: Paula, who also betrays Harry), and destructive bad breasts (Arlene's silicone-boosted breasts); the place of Harry's mother in this split remains enigmatic. When Harry finds Delly (Melanie Griffith), she too initially appears as a dangerous temptress (her full name is Delilah), and her seductiveness towards him is also expressed by baring her breasts; but with her he appears embarrassed, and turns his head away.

Harry's growing affection towards Delly, most evident after her nightmare, is tender, parental and non-incestuous. When he holds her to calm her down, she talks about feeling 'before you were born, your mother's heart beating on your back'. His identification with her is striking. 'Did you ever run away from home?' she asks, and he jokes: 'Me and my parents, we had a different arrangement'. He appears to know that these 'arrangements' are inherently similar: Delly was practically abandoned by her father, and his money appears to be the main reason why her mother wants her back home. Arlene has always been more involved with her lovers than with her daughter, and Delly's escape from home is accompanied by repeated efforts to seduce her mother's former lovers, including Delly's ex-stepfather Tom (John Crawford). Indeed, Harry manages to locate her in Tom's house in the Florida Keys thanks to a dynamic, oedipal interpretation: 'Maybe she is trying to even up the score'.

Ellen: 'It has taken us a long time to get this far, I don't want to pour it all away. Please.'

We could ironically speak of 'the two analyses of Delly G'. The first 'analysis' takes place while Harry is being betrayed by his wife. His mute expression when first seeing Ellen with Marty is a vivid depiction of painful primal scene affects. This personal preoccupation is part of Harry's 'countertransference' in analysing Delly's case, and contributes to his focus on interpreting oedipal dynamics. This first analysis is seemingly successful: Harry is able to help Delly renounce her incestuous affair with her former stepfather, and return home. But homecoming deteriorates into a violent row, and Harry appears shaken by the sarcastic confrontation of Delly's boyfriend Quentin (James Woods): 'Are you satisfied? You got another happy family together'.

When learning later of Delly's violent death, Harry must reconsider his understanding. The second part of the film is a 'second analysis', in search of the fuller truth, external and internal. Harry is reunited with Ellen, and starts grappling with questions he evaded before: 'the identity of his wife, his relation to her, his relation to his father, his identity, who he is and what he is' (Penn, in Gallagher, 1975, p. 87). He is now able to see that his oedipal-sexual focus (a partially correct but insufficient interpretation) may have blinded him to Delly's plight as a rejected child; and in returning Delly to her mother he may have actually colluded in her exploitation by her mother (repeating Delly's past injuries rather than curing them as he wished), and endangered her life.

Harry's rage towards destructive parenting mounts. 'Delly had no chance with you as a mother, she was on a downhill flight right from the start', he screams at Arlene in their last furious encounter. Arlene bitterly answers: 'Delly wasn't the only kid who ever had it rough'. We may be reminded of the gunshot suicide committed by Arlene's father (when she was 8); but this casual early bit of information remains in the background, and Arlene never gains our empathy.

Harry's guilt towards both Delly and Ellen preoccupies him in his second, more daring and more penetrating search. In going again to Florida, he abandons Ellen once more. But the two parting scenes are markedly different. In the first, each of them is in another car, and Harry angrily rushes to go, refusing to talk with Ellen who begs him to stay for one more day. In the second, Ellen accompanies him to the airport, he explains to her why it is crucial for him to go and figure out the truth, and promises to be back 'no later than Friday'. He tells her affectionately: 'I know you have been alone a lot, even when I was around. And I know when you get ... when we get like that we reach out for other people'. Offering Ellen an empathic interpretation, he also remorsefully hints at his affair with Paula; and in switching to 'we' he acknowledges his and Ellen's common anguish. Earlier on, when Ellen used the word 'we', Harry exploded with projective moralistic blaming. The change of outlook and of tone is striking, as after a successful working through of a painful experience.

Although Ellen is visibly sad and worried, she also probes him not to miss his plane, saying: 'If you don't go now, you can't come back'. While made jokingly, this comment seems to convey her awareness that solving his 'inner detective story' is for Harry a crucial step towards forming a more real relationship with her. This too is an empathic interpretation, recognising the different meaning of Harry's present departure in comparison to his driven disappearances so far. And while many scenes in this film are cut short, contributing to its unsettling effect, in this scene the camera lingers attentively on lonely Ellen after Harry boards his plane. We know she wants him back.

The final sequence in Florida is very intense. Harry discovers that Tom, Paula and Quentin were all part of a ring smuggling precious antiques from the Yucatan, and that Delly was probably murdered after she discovered their plots. At the end of a bloody trail, an aeroplane appears, Harry is shot and wounded, Paula is killed, and when the plane drowns Harry recognises the face of the dying pilot: his older friend and confidant, the charming stuntman Joey Ziegler (Edward Binns). Joey attempts to talk to Harry, but through the drowning plane's thick windowpane only his lips are seen moving, like those of Harry's father when he finally traced him years ago. The discovery that fatherly Joey was the ringleader, possibly had killed Delly, and attempted to kill Harry, brings us full circle to the initial betrayal by the father.

Wounded Harry manages to start the engine of his boat (called *'Point of View'*), but cannot steer it, and the scene fades out with the boat going around in circles. For me, however, there is a shred of hope in this bleak ending: the fantasy that Harry can be discovered and brought to shore, allowed to recover at Ellen's bosom.

Paula (watching Harry's chess manoeuvre): 'It's a beauty!'

Harry: 'But he didn't see it. He played something else, and he lost. Must have regretted it every day of his life. I know so would I. In fact, I do regret it, and I wasn't born yet.'

Paula: 'That's no excuse.'

Harry is in many ways an heir to Hammett's Sam Spade (Marty challenges Harry to hit him, 'the way Sam Spade would'), just as the precious antique is a variation on the phallic Maltese Falcon. Loyal to the Hammett–Chandler–Macdonald image of the detective, he is violent, sexual and troubled himself, and yet an uncompromising truth-seeker.

But the film markedly differs from genre traditions. While *The Maltese Falcon* 'is completely devoid of any explicit reference to inner feeling states or motives' (Bauer et al., 1978, p. 283), *Night Moves* is psychologically minded and often interpretive. While Spade and similar protagonists maintain a detached cynical view of self and others, Harry Mosby evolves out of that position, acquiring insightful and empathic capacities. And while women in most *noir* detective stories and films remain two-dimensional, and

Spade's final victory signifies 'asserting his invulnerability to the seductive powers of [deceitful] Brigid' (Bauer et al., 1997, p. 294), Ellen represents a possibility of overcoming splits and projections, of integrating sexuality and companionship, vulnerability and strength.

These unique aspects of *Night Moves* make a purely oedipal understanding (the detective as an aroused, inquisitive oedipal child; see Bauer et al., 1978) insufficient. There are strong oedipal motives and primal scene allusions (including the film's name), but they are better understood in a broader context of object relations and self-development. Being an unwelcome child ('regretting every day of his life what happened before he was born') underlies Harry's oedipal conflict; his incapacity to handle the triangular situation ('he didn't see it ... and he lost') stems from his despair about dyadic relations, preventing him from full relatedness to a woman, as well as from parenthood.

Reliving—through Delly's tragedy—his childhood abandonment, re-experiencing his rage, gaining insight into repetition-compulsion in his work and personal life, and rediscovering Ellen's devotion, enable Harry to grow. The film follows him through pain and disillusion, but allows him new vistas, and therefore some hope.

REFERENCES

BAUER, S. F. ET AL. (1978). The detective film as myth: *The Maltese Falcon* and Sam Spade. *Amer. Imago*, 35: 275-296.

BERMAN, E. (1997). Hitchcock's *Vertigo*: the collapse of a rescue fantasy. *Int. J. Psychoanal.*, 78: 975-996.

—— (1998). The film viewer: from dreamer to dream interpreter. *Psychoanal. Inq.*, 18: 193-206.

GALLAGHER, T. (1975). *Night Moves. Sight & Sound,* 44: 86-90.

SIMON, B. (1985). 'With cunning delays and evermounting excitement': or, what thickens the plot in psychoanalysis and tragedy? In *Psychoanalysis: The Vital Issues, Vol. 2,* ed. J. Gedo & G. Pollock. New York: Int. Univ. Press, pp. 387-435.

8. *LONE STAR*:
SIGNS, BORDERS AND THRESHOLDS

HARRIET KIMBLE WRYE, Pacific Palisades

In *Lone Star*, written, directed and edited by John Sayles (1995), hidden and evocative bits and pieces of characters' lives emerge and are interwoven, as in an analysis. Past and present are never divided by uncrossable borders; porosity of the mind is dramatically realised in Sayles's seamless editing, shifting from one temporal perspective in a character's inner world to another. At the same time, however, Sayles describes his film as a 'story about borders', which he defines not only geographically, setting the film in the mythical Frontera, Texas (the town's name actually means border in Spanish), but psychologically as well: 'A border is where you draw a line and say, "This is where I end and somebody else begins"' (West, 1997, p. 14). Sayles is interested in the lines drawn between people—sex, class, race, age. In this review, I also propose that he is interested in thresholds and epiphanic border crossings, if you will, that permit a dialectic whereby a rigid point of demarcation may be transformed. These 'thresholds' occur in dramatic moments within the film and between the film screen and the audience.

The film's serious theme, often comically underscored, is about the deformative social constructions of power, race, age and gender. Sayles's cinematic eye draws our attention to his theme through

visual images: signs of proprietorship, borders, military rank, gender, race, signs evoking prejudice. The logo of the film, the Texas
sheriff's 'lone star' badge, is a sign both of political power and corruption and decay. Projections of idealisation or devaluation are
represented via the abandoned drive-in film screen, formerly the
site of such projections. The barren Texas landscape of *Lone Star* is
dotted with signs, actual and symbolic, signifying borders of all
kinds—incestual, metonymic, interpersonal, ideological, geograph-
ical, political, racial and gendered. As well as portraying certain
psychic rigidities associated with primitive mental states, *Lone Star*
can also be read as a text on transformational border crossings.

BORDERS

As prohibitors and separators, we associate borders with barbed-
wire fences, the Berlin Wall, the Great Wall of China, and dangerous, often fatal, crossings such as the Rio Grande. Much of the
haunting power of *Lone Star* lies in its evocative study of various
kinds of border crossings. John Sayles once said, 'I remember [a]
film ... and the last scene is of this woman who's been waiting by
the border, crossing five feet into the U.S. side and handcuffing herself to a pole before giving birth so her kid will be an American
citizen ... that's some heavy shit. She moved from here to there and
all of a sudden her kid is another person' (West, 1997, p. 15).

The film's infamous Sheriff Charlie Wade (Kris Kristofferson),
like an attack dog, viciously patrolled the Mexican border. He
ruthlessly shot Eladio Cruz, Mercedes's husband, for aiding ille-

gal aliens. Corrupt to the bone, Wade was a specialist in 'La Mor-
dida' which is what Mexicans call payola or extortion. In this
sense, Wade carries Sayles's theme that rigidity of authority leads
to a kind of corruption and spiritual annihilation, a collapsing of
meaning. The film's opening image of Wade's skull and badge
rusting in the desert evoke a Bergmanesque *Seventh Seal* icon of
the mortification of the flesh and the vanity of vanities, God's final
punishment for greed, cruelty and sadism: 'Across that line you're
Sheriff of nothing'.

Lone Star deals with the boundaries between generations—parents, children and grandchildren, and is rich with oedipal themes
and incestual crossings. 'Lone Star' also refers to son Sam's need to
differentiate himself from his valorised 'star' father, Sheriff Buddy,
who also betrayed his 'sainted' mother. The father–son dramatic
line is represented by Buddy (Matthew McConaughey) and Sam
Deeds (Chris Cooper), Otis (Ron Canada) and Delmar Payne (Joe
Morton) and Payne's adolescent boy, Chet; the mother–child dra-
mas are carried by Mercedes (Miriam Colon), her daughter Pilar
Cruz (Elizabeth Pena) and Pilar's children.

Sayles repeatedly illustrates how unyielding mental borders
reflect a primitive mental state, Freud's purified pleasure principle
or Klein's paranoid position (1975)—where everything that is on
the other side is bad, 'not me' and to be warded off. Sayles portrays
such rigidity as a defence against fears of abandonment and inade-
quacy, as in the former wetback Mercedes Cruz's insistence that all
Mexicans 'Speak English!' and in the character structure of Colonel
Delmar Payne (Joe Morton), an alienated 'real hard case. A spit and
polish man' who, it turns out, has hardened himself to cover over the

wounds of what he felt was his father Otis's early abandonment. So he becomes a reified caricature of dying paternalism, top dog on an army base he is there to terminate. Rigid mental and physical border patrolling is contrasted with moral integrity exercised by individuals making mindful choices.

Such personal ethical choices, however, may leave one isolated outside conventional borders and are embodied by disenfranchised subjects such as Eladio Cruz, brutally sacrificed by Sheriff Wade; the independent-minded Indian trading-post owner Sam visits on the 'stretch of road between nowhere and not much else' and pivotally by half-sibling lovers Pilar and Sam, choosing to inhabit the no-man's-land outside the incest barrier. This takes us to the third area of my title, *thresholds*. In contrast to borders that differentiate, contain, limit and circumscribe, thresholds are passageways meant to be crossed, and imply entrances, beginnings and openings.

THRESHOLDS

In an article honouring the centennial of film and psychoanalysis, Judith Welles (1998) has posited that a threshold may be understood as a particular kind of narrative space (see also Wrye & Welles, 1994), which requires a new logic and a perspective beyond conventional orders of causality, sequence and selection: '[Thresholds] sponsor the consideration of dialectics. A threshold is a particular, often ephemeral, set of consciousness, in which the limits of familiar sameness and reputed difference are extended and enriched by holding simultaneously in mind a glimpse of the other and of the self ... This new way is ... transitional in the sense of promoting change, and it is epigenetic in the sense that it has never existed in either culture ... Such original products may prove momentary or lasting, depending on the course of events' (1998, p. 217).

John Sayles, I believe, would like Welles's notion, for I think he offers several such thresholds in this film, where we see a character move from a potentially closed border, an intransigent position, to an opening of the mind, in a transformational experience. Such a moment occurs for Colonel Delmar Payne, when he opens himself enough literally to cross the threshold of his estranged father's house. Crossing this threshold offers him the opportunity to see something that has always been there, but that he has been too cut off to see. Namely, that his father adores him, is proud of him, and has been saving every news clipping heralding his son's career. The Colonel realises that he has been operating since childhood under the notion that his father didn't care about him, an archaic narrative fed to him by his hurt and jealous mother. But this was *her* vindictive narrative, and not the truth. Payne had been preparing himself for such a moment by questioning the rigidity of his military values. He moves to this threshold moment in the earlier scene where, as base commander, he is to discipline a young black female private for drug use. Asking her why she joined the army, she ingenuously offers him the truth instead of patriotic pap: 'It's the best job they got'. And, she adds, they 'let us in on this deal 'cause *they* gotta have somebody to fight the Arabs and yellow people ... Might as well be *us* (*sic* blacks), Sir?' This, plus Payne's own adolescent son's quest for a different sort of father more like his grandfather who teaches him the proud black history of the Seminoles, sets Payne to questioning many of his assumptions. In this sense for Payne it is a 'painful' threshold where one's unstated assumptions are made salient, and held up to comparison with the unstated assumptions of the other. This new way is both transitional and epigenetic (Welles, 1998).

At the same time, Sayles cautions us that such border transcendencies may offer personal freedom, but they do not fundamentally change the society against which they are exercised. The fact that this love cannot produce children gives it an acceptability that is totally different from the corrupt incestual relationship in *Angels and Insects*, which wreaked havoc on a marriage and produced monster progeny, or the ingrown incestuousness portrayed in the family in *Hotel New Hampshire*. Moreover, we sense that Pilar and Sam will have to leave Frontera to live together, that they cannot change the entrenched public opinion of their home town.

This brings me to my concluding point about how thresholds function in relation to film and audience like the intermediate or transitional space between analyst and analysand. This third area in film viewing may be conceptualised by marrying Kristeva's 'privileged moment' (1980), Bollas's 'aesthetic moment' (1993), Sanville's 'analytic playground' (1991), my own descriptions of 'narrative space' (1994; Wrye & Welles, 1994), Ogden's 'analytic third' (1994a, b), and Welles's 'threshold' (1998). Space exists between filmmaker, film and audience, providing a playground for creative transformation. This intermediate or transitional space relates to Winnicott's 'neither inside nor outside' (1952) which Königsberg (1996) has recently related to film spectatorship. The film-maker offers his conscious and unconscious communications dramatically and imagistically. In the case of a poetic film like *Lone Star*, the ripples in the pools of the audience's conscious and unconscious mind are deeply stirred by these images. Regressed, sunken in soft plush velvet in the darkened theatre, like an analytic reverie, the audience, open to a reverberating dialectical process within this 'cinematic third area', is receptive to moving 'outside the individual domain of the two ongoing narratives it situates' (film-maker's and viewer's preconceptions) to 'articulate the fissure between them' (Welles, 1998, p. 217), thereby creating a threshold, extending the boundaries of the viewer's psyche, and sponsoring a dialectic process, which, according to Ogden, is: 'a process in which opposing elements each create, preserve, and negate each other; each stands in a dynamic, ever-changing relationship to the other ... Each potential integration creates a new form of opposition characterised by its own distinct form of dialectical tension' (1994a, p. 14).

In this sense, while certain townspeople in mythical Frontera are frozen, captured in celluloid clinging rigidly to their borders, *Lone Star*'s viewing audience may be caught up in the dialectic, brought to a threshold and transformed. We are invited to move from narrow dichotomised paradigms to embrace the view that Otis Payne, the Mayor of Darktown, sponsors: 'It's not like there's a borderline between the good people and the bad people—you're not on one side or the other'. Even as psychoanalysts we are brought by Sayles to a threshold on which we can consider incest from a different vantage point.

REFERENCES

BOLLAS, C. (1993). The aesthetic moment and the search for transformation. In *Transitional Objects and Potential Spaces: Literary Uses of D. W. Winnicott*, ed. P. Rudnytsky. New York: Columbia Univ. Press, pp. 40-49.

KLEIN, M. (1975). *Love, Guilt and Reparation and Other Works, 1921-1945.* New York: Delacorte.

KÖNIGSBERG, I. (1996). Transitional phenomena, transitional space: creativity and spectatorship in film. *Psychoanal. Rev.*, 83: 865-890.

KRISTEVA, J. (1980). *Desire in Language.* New York: Columbia Univ. Press.

OGDEN, T. A. (1994a). *Subjects of Analysis.* New Jersey: Jason Aronson.

—— (1994b). The analytic third—working with intersubjective facts. *Int. J. Psychoanal.*, 75: 3-20.

SANVILLE, J. (1991). *The Playground of Psychoanalytic Therapy.* Hillsdale, NJ: The Analytic Press.

WELLES, J. K. (1998). Rituals: cinematic and analytic. *Psychoanal. Inq.*, Centennial issue on film and psychoanalysis (ed. H. K. Wrye & D. Diamond), 18: 207-221.

WEST, D. J. (1997). Borders and boundaries: an interview with John Sayles. *Cinéaste*, 26: 14-17.

WINNICOTT, D. W. (1952). Transitional objects and transitional phenomena. In *Playing and Reality*. New York: Basic Books, pp. 38-57.

WRYE, H. K. (1994). Narrative scripts: composing a life with ambition and desire. *Amer. J. Psychoanal.*, 54: 127-142.

—— & WELLES, J. K. (1994). *The Narration of Desire: Erotic Transference and Countertransference.* Hillsdale, NJ: The Analytic Press.

9. LETTERS, WORDS AND METAPHORS: A PSYCHOANALYTIC READING OF MICHAEL RADFORD'S *IL POSTINO*

ANDREA SABBADINI, London

'WANTED—POSTMAN WITH BICYCLE.' Only a temporary job, but almost tailor-made for Mario (Massimo Troisi), an introverted and uneducated yet sharply insightful young man, protagonist of Michael Radford's delightfully bitter-sweet, humane, humorous, moving yet never sentimental comedy *Il Postino.* The job involves carrying the mail to just one illustrious addressee, the Chilean poet Pablo Neruda (Philippe Noiret) exiled in the early 1950s to the Southern Italian island of Procida because of his communist views. Every day Mario pedals up to the poet's new residence—a villa located on the top of a hill, surrounded by wild Mediterranean vegetation and overlooking the sea—carrying a leather bag full of correspondence: mostly, at least in his adolescent mind fuelled by newsreel mythology, love letters from adoring women all over the world.

At first, of course, Mario and Neruda hardly talk. What is there to be said, anyway, between them? Intrigued by his own thoughts and feelings, the postman cannot find the words to express them and the poet has better things to do than listen to him. But, as the relationship develops, Mario finds an interlocutor and, with it, a voice: tentative at first, when he dares, after a farcical rehearsal in front of the mirror, to ask the poet for an autograph in the hope that this will impress his girlfriends in Naples—then progressively more secure. In Neruda-the-Man he gradually discovers the parental figure to identify with and idealise; in Neruda-the-Poet the language to make sense of his inner world. If Mario's real father is a silent, down-to-earth (or down-to-sea) fisherman with little understanding of his son's existential problems ('I am tired of being a man', Mario says echoing Neruda's words), his dead mother is entirely absent—other than, that is, in the guises of Nature, both literally in the external world, and literarily in Neruda's, and then Mario's own, poetry: an all-embracing, all-containing and nurturing sea surrounding the beautiful—part lush, part desert—island.

The film has the structure, familiar to fiction readers and cinema-goers alike, of a *Bildungsroman*. Witnessed by the poet himself, Mario's development into a mature man culminates in his achievement of potency, which finds its expression at three different, but interconnected, levels: (1) *sexual* through his relationship, as passionate as it is clumsy, to maidenly sensuous waitress Beatrice (Maria Grazia Cucinotta), whom he eventually marries, with Neruda's help and blessing; (2) *literary* as Mario starts reading and producing verse himself, and even suggesting to his own Master an excellent adjective ('sad') to describe what fishing-nets look like. It is not a coincidence that he will unself-consciously create his first metaphor when listening to Neruda's lyrical description of the sea: 'I feel ... weird and seasick', he says, 'like a boat tossing around ... WORDS'; and finally (3) *political* by tentatively opposing a local Mafioso boss and through an ill-fated involvement with a communist demonstration, where he is invited to read one of his own Neruda-inspired poems to the crowd.

Part of the fascination of *Il Postino* consists in creatively immers-
ing a real and contemporary character, the poet Pablo Neruda here
portrayed with much biographical accuracy, in an entirely fictional
situation. But if the filmmaker's fantasy interplays with history, the
external world also intrudes, and most tragically, into the artistic
work: as soon as the shooting of *Il Postino* was over Massimo Troisi,
the actor in the title role, prematurely died. In the film, Mario is
killed at a mass rally during an incident with the police: a conclusion
perhaps ideological and aesthetically unnecessary, but also providing the viewers who are aware of Troisi's death with a powerfully
unheimlich experience of life imitating art.

I would like to suggest here that Neruda is also Mario's 'psychoanalyst'. The 'sessions' are represented by the postman's uphill
journeys by bicycle, at regular intervals, to the poet's villa. Such
ritualised visits, charged as they are for Mario with meaningful
words and silences, half-monologues and half-dialogues, readily
become opportunities for him to learn about love, literature, relationships and, ultimately, himself. A central mechanism in this 'therapeutic' process is identification: 'I'd like to be a poet too', says
Mario, and asks Neruda how to become one—a wish that the latter
only superficially discourages ('You'll get as fat as me!'). The post-
man/patient identifies with the poet/analyst: his wish to become
like him is so frequent in clinical practice that it could be hyperboli-
cally argued that, in fantasy at least, all analyses are training analyses!

Mario's journeys to the poet's villa, at the same time, are also
more regressive explorations of 'primal scene' unconscious fantasies, as exemplified by the love letters he delivers, and is explicitly

curious about, to Neruda as well as by the poet's openly sensual relationship with his wife Matilde. The first time Mario finds them hugging he modestly hides away. Later however, after he has himself established a sexual relationship with Beatrice, he allows himself some vicarious pleasure by watching the Nerudas dance a passionate tango.

We can recognise a number of important elements, crucial to the film's narrative and characterisations, which are also integral aspects of the psychoanalytic experience. For example, our postman alternates between blaming Neruda for his love problems with Beatrice and expecting him to resolve them—a situation not unfamiliar to psychoanalysts. The name Beatrice is itself evocative, being also the name of the woman who inspired Dante Alighieri, whose presence in the background as the Father of all Poets reminds one of the part played in many analyses by Sigmund Freud, the Father of all Psychoanalysts. (Neruda and Freud, by the way, were both candidates, though only the former successfully, for the Nobel Prize— and *Il Postino* for five Academy awards.)

Neruda tells Mario that 'poetry is the experience of feeling', a statement that could as well apply to psychoanalysis: indeed, they both provide alternative perspectives on the world—and a language to describe it. It is significant, I think, that our hero is a postman, he who 'carries across' ('transfers') emotionally loaded messages, and that his conversations with the poet often revolve around the subject of 'metaphors', a word that in the film becomes itself a metaphor for all that is not prosaic in life. It is after all primarily through their interpretive work, which depends on such rhetorical devices as metaphors and analogies, that analysts help analysands understand the complex connections between different sets of thoughts, emotions and relationships. Furthermore, having the same etymology as 'transference', the concept of metaphor seems ideal to indicate the associations between literature and psychoanalysis and, in its audio and visual representations, cinema itself. Words—the stuff both poetry and 'the talking cure' are made of—are powerful. Even Beatrice's bigoted, but not idiotic, Aunt Rosa, constantly worried about her niece's virginity, can state that 'a man is not far off with his hands when he starts touching you with his words!'

Of course, Neruda's 'countertransference' relationship to Mario—as he has always suspected, but also denied until its reality becomes overwhelmingly painful—is coloured by ambivalence, and not just or even primarily because of its homosexual undertones: the poet, at least in Mario's projective fantasies, is partly the benevolent parental figure we assume he has never had, partly the detached, indifferent, cold professional—almost a caricature of a psychoanalyst—ready to forget him as soon as the 'contract' is over, as soon as he can return to Chile and there is no more correspondence to be delivered. When Neruda embraces Mario before leaving the island, the 'termination' of their relationship is as deeply felt by both of them as the one at the end of a good analysis. 'You left something behind for me!' says Mario, who is now ready to internalise the poet/father/analyst and get on with life on his own, though of course not without much sadness. But then his mentor fails to keep in touch: when at long last, after more than one year, Mario receives a letter from Chile, it is a disappointingly impersonal message from the poet's secretary, asking for some effects left behind in the by now dilapidated villa to be returned. Mario feels devastated but still tries to rationalise the poet's behaviour: 'Why should he remember me? … I think it's quite normal', he says … but with bitter tears in his eyes.

Michael Radford's *Il Postino* may not be what is conventionally understood as a 'psychoanalytic' film. Attempting to interpret the unconscious meanings of an exiled communist poet's behaviour and verse, or of an islander's everyday life preoccupations, would have been a futile exercise; the film has minimal symbolism in its imagery, no dream sequences, no scenes taking place in a mental institution or in a therapist's consulting room, no display of violence, perversion or psychopathology. And yet the description of a process of maturation through an intense personal rapport full of transference and countertransference connotations, which is central to this movie, has much in common, in its structure and function, with the psychoanalytic relationship. In this respect, viewing *Il Postino* through a psychoanalytic lens by drawing parallels between the two situations will hopefully enrich and deepen our understanding of both.

10. TRUFFAUT AND THE FAILURE OF INTROJECTION

SIMONA ARGENTIERI, ROME

My reflections are on two films by François Truffaut: *L'homme qui aimait les femmes* ('The Man Who Loved Women', 1977) and *La chambre verte* ('The Green Room', 1978), produced within a year of each other. At a first viewing, they seem to be two very different works. *La chambre verte*, dramatic and painful, is based on a sombre short story by Henry James, 'The Altar of the Dead', and on two other of his works, 'The Beast in the Jungle' and 'The Friends of Friends'. It is the story of Julian Davenne, a 'virtuoso' in necrology, and his passionate loving obsession for one woman alone—his wife who died young—even after her death and until his own death. The other film, *L'homme qui aimait les femmes*, is a delightfully ironic comedy of the autobiographical type, in which the protagonist continually falls in love with every woman he meets, and in which there is the hint of a delightful touch of foot and leg fetishism.

Both films, however, in spite of the great differences in language, style and narrative, basically tell the same story of the incapacity to love and to make one's own internal impulse coincide with the encounter with a real person. The protagonist of *L'homme qui aimait les femmes* does not know how to distinguish or to choose, in a giddy erotic round of seduction, unfaithfulness and disillusion in which the illusion is repeatedly rekindled. In *La chambre verte*, Julian is imprisoned in a repetitive trap of an opposite kind. Tenaciously faithful to the image of one woman alone, he cannot conceive of a love object unless it is eternally identical to itself. Whether in a state of immobility or in flight, both characters are living outside of real time, enslaved by an obsession.

In *La chambre verte*, Truffaut's outstanding intuition lies in showing us how the impossibility of completing the mourning process coincides with the impossibility of loving. The drama of Julian Davenne, a kind of 'platonic' necrophile, is not so much the sorrow of having lost his real wife; it is the suffering caused by not being able to keep his love for her alive within himself, and his fear of losing the remembrance of her, of being unable to keep her image in his mind. The many photographs and portraits with which he surrounds himself are fragile, inadequate substitutes for the memory, and his obsessive worship of them is the symptom of the precariousness of his internal symbolic world. This is dramatically illustrated by the grotesque failure of the wax figure that he tries to make as a 'faithful' copy of his dead wife, but that turns out to be only a useless fetish. Or in the scene of his first conversation with Cecilie, the woman who tries to bring him back to love and to life as she tenderly recalls their first meeting long ago, while he—who lives in the cult of the past—remembers nothing.

We know that the making of a film is a collective effort, and it is therefore arbitrary to try to identify the author in the director alone. But in these two films, the choice of subject, the scenario, the role of actor in the first film and the obvious autobiographical references in the second would seem to authorise us to explore the interweavings between the artist's internal vicissitudes, his statements in books and interviews, and the expressive quality of the film 'texts'. Thus, I think it is particularly interesting to note the changes that Truffaut makes in the film version, beginning with the change in title from the lugubrious 'The Altar of the Dead' to *La chambre verte*. In spite of the authentic suffering that pervades it, the film is full of emotions of intense sensuality.

In my view, there are two changes that are the most significant. One is the introduction of the deaf-mute boy—apparently so incoherent in the development of events. This impaired but vibrant image seems to be a self-quotation from *L'enfant sauvage* (1969) in which Truffaut, as he did in *La chambre verte*, chose to play the part of the main character, Professor Itard, who tries in vain to bring the little wolf-boy back into the human community.[1] Truffaut wrote: 'It seemed to me that if I myself played the part of Julien Davenne, I would obtain the same difference as when ... I decide to write certain of my letters directly by hand'. To me, this seems to indicate the profound consonance of Truffaut—ex 'wild' boy—with all his tender rebellious and misunderstood childhood, and this is certainly one of the most moving themes of his whole cinematographic production. Young George in *La chambre verte* who first breaks (the

---

[1] Cinema fans will have noticed another 'quotation' in the absurd episode of the child in prison, in which Truffaut reproduces on the screen a childhood recollection of Alfred Hitchcock who talks about it in his well-known published interview. With the connivance of a friend in the police force, Hitchcock's father had him shut in a prison cell for a few minutes 'to teach him a lesson'. 'But what had you done to deserve such a punishment?', asks Truffaut. 'I haven't the slightest idea' is the reply (Truffaut, 1983).

photographic slides, the shop window in order to steal the wax dummy, once again a female image!), and who then repairs (the projector, helping to repair the chapel etc.), demonstrates the infantile antecedents not only of Davenne but of Truffaut himself; an infancy marked by solitude, desperation, unconscious guilt and innocence.

The second element introduced by Truffaut that confers meaning and depth to the whole story is precisely this feeling of guilt; the guilt of the one who has survived and cannot accept the injustice not only of the premature death of his wife, but also of the hundreds of soldiers killed in the war as a result of human destructiveness. Truffaut's great artistic intuition lies precisely in this dimension of anguish and guilt combined with the theme of hatred and of impossible forgiveness for his old friend now dead—a dimension also present in the original story by Henry James. In fact, at the beginning of the film, the images that run behind the titles are original documentaries of the First World War.

In the scene of the chapel, where Davenne celebrates the cult of his deceased wife and of all his other beloved dead, scenario and biography overlap as the camera, in the expert hands of Nestor Almendros, skims lightly over the portraits of the dead in the candle-lit gallery. Davenne's dead are Truffaut's dead, intermingled with the portraits of his favourite authors—Henry James himself, Cocteau, Wilde, Proust, Balzac—in a kind of affective equivalence between books and people. (This brings to mind the little altar that the child Antoine Doinel erects in memory of Balzac in *Les 400 coups* (1959), and also Truffaut who surrounded himself with photos of his friends together with those of the film directors of the past). But in this gallery of the dead, there is an even more disquieting and revealing image. In the uniform of a German soldier, Truffaut has put the photo of Oscar Werner, still alive at that time, who had acted for him in *Jules et Jim* and in *Fahrenheit 451*, and with whom he had shared a passionate friendship and then an irremediable dispute. 'I am one of his murderers', says Davenne.

In *L'homme qui aimait les femmes*, one of the many variations on the autobiographical theme after *Les 400 coups*, *Antoine et Colette*, *Baisers volés*, *Domicile conjugale*, etc., we see the protagonist, Bertrand, desperately and permanently in love but always with a different woman. By now he is well past his youth, but he continues becoming entranced, letting himself be seduced and then abandoning, always with the same cruel innocence. In a brief but revealing flashback we see him as a small child, sitting on the floor. The camera moves at the level of his eyes that are focused on the legs of his mother while she paces backwards and forwards threateningly, scolding him for some unspecified misdeeds. While Davenne was condemned to the worship of one woman alone, Bertrand loves and hates them all because they are interchangeable and repetitive objects that construct nothing inside him. They are all equivalent because they all disappoint him in the play of illusion, like so many anonymous mirrors in which he only fleetingly catches a glimpse of his own reflection. When fate leads him to meet the only woman he has really loved again, he does not recognise her, just as Davenne did not remember Cecilie. Unable to construct an authentic relationship, Bertrand flees before his anxiety, using every euphoric and manic defence and putting Eros at the service of the compulsion to repeat. Julian, on the other hand, has accepted with complete transparency to face the very core of his depressive anxiety. Using his own countenance in the part of Julian, without even the mediation of an actor, Truffaut lives the sense of death, solitude and the absence of love. If defensive desires rather than authentic needs are satisfied, then resistance towards comprehension and symbolisation is reinforced and the only destiny remaining is that of the repetition compulsion, by acting out what cannot be thought or remembered or symbolised.

In conclusion, I think that these two films enable us to explore the links between artistic creativity and life and to understand, with the help of the extraordinary expressive capacity of this author, those universal human vicissitudes that psychoanalysis explores. It seems to me that through his films, Truffaut describes for us and for himself his childhood drama of not having had a symbolic space in the internal world of his mother or—in symmetry with this —the possibility of constructing within himself a safe and stable image of the female figure. Perhaps by continually running away from home, the child François (as well as his film characters) was trying to make his parents perceive his absence. Perhaps it is in order to follow this poetic reasoning of his that in spite of the considerable formal differences between *La chambre verte* and *L'homme qui aimait les femmes* Truffaut decided to end both of them with the death of the protagonist.

It is remarkable that it should be a man of the cinema who tells us about this drama of obsession with images; someone who by vocation and unconscious motivations is able to capture, evoke, create and re-create by means of the camera all the images of his own internal reality. For, through psychoanalysis, we have come to understand that art—for those who create it as well as for those who enjoy it—is not only 'consolation' but also 'reparation'; it is an attempt to repair what, in the past, has been lost or damaged in our internal world.[2] Perhaps it is for this reason that Truffaut says: 'This is why I am the happiest of men: I fulfil all my dreams and I am paid for doing it. I am a film director'.

Reference

Truffaut, F. (1983). *Le cinéma selon Hitchcock.* Paris: Éditions Ramsay.

---

[2] In his 1983 re-make of *The Man Who Loved Women,* Blake Edwards has caught this aspect of psychoanalytical elaboration, although in a superficial and somewhat banal manner, by transferring the story of Bertrand to the psychoanalyst's couch.

11. I HAVE NOT SPOKEN: SILENCE IN *THE PIANO*

BRUCE H. SKLAREW, Chevy Chase, MD

In Jane Campion's *The Piano*, Ada (Holly Hunter) meets Stewart
(Sam Neill), her husband by an arranged marriage, on a beach full of
foreboding in the dream-like wilderness of mid-nineteenth-century
New Zealand. Arriving by ship from Scotland, she has waited over-
night with her 9-year-old daughter, Flora. Her most precious possession, a piano, is left on the beach by the awkward and unempathic
Stewart. It is later rescued by Baines (Harvey Keitel), another set-
tler, in an exchange for land with Stewart. Feigning interest in
piano lessons from Ada, Baines offers to return the piano to her in
exchange for sexual favours. Eventually they fall in love. When
Flora reveals to Stewart that her mother's affair continues, Stewart
chops off part of Ada's finger. Having relinquished hope of gaining
Ada's love, Stewart allows Ada and Flora to leave with Baines, and
they establish a family.

This voice-over accompanies establishing shots of Ada's life in
Scotland before her journey to New Zealand.

> The voice you hear is not my speaking voice, but my mind's voice.
> I have not spoken since I was 6 years old. No one
> knows why, not even me. My father says it is a dark talent and the day
> I take it into my head to stop breathing will be my last.
>
> Today he married me to a man I've not yet met.
> Soon my daughter and I shall join him in his own

country. My husband said my muteness does not
bother him. He writes, and hark this: God loves dumb creatures,
so why not he. Were good he had God's patience, for silence
affects everyone in the end. The strange thing
is I don't think myself silent, that is, because
of my piano. I shall miss it on the journey.

A notable quality of *The Piano* is the dearth of information about Ada's childhood other than the sudden onset of her muteness at the age of 6. There is no mention of her mother. But director Jane Campion's powerful visual imagery mobilises our conscious and unconscious fantasies to suggest links between present and past. These images convey the themes of abandonment and primal scene trauma, and suggest the origins of Ada's muteness.

In the film we see multiple representations of the merged and interchangeable identities of Ada and Flora. Flora speaks for Ada, and Campion presents many two-shots of Ada and Flora in the same pose with heads similarly tilted. Flora resonates to her mother's mood and appearance.

We know that parents often re-live traumatic childhood events by unconsciously inflicting the same or similar experiences upon their children, turning passive into active. Flora views the primal scene in Baines's cabin, perhaps unconsciously 'arranged' by her mother. And her mother brings her into her love life by using her as a messenger to carry a piano key with a love message to Baines (that instead she gives to Stewart) just as later Stewart orders her to take the piece of Ada's finger to Baines. Although Ada doesn't orchestrate it, Flora, nevertheless, is subjected to the horror of watching the amputation of part of Ada's finger, a primal scene equivalent.

Flora's jarring cartoon-like fantasy of a lightning bolt causing the death of her father and the muteness of her mother as they are singing in the Pyrenees combines the primal scene, muteness, destructiveness and death. The viewer, using Flora's experience, supplies missing links to Ada's past and muteness and could imagine that Ada might have viewed a powerful primal scene such as a forbidden sexual liaison. The viewer might further fantasise that, like Flora, a revelation by Ada might have had unexpected violent consequences. Ada could have feared that if words can be dangerous, it is safer to be mute. But Ada's love message on the piano key is a transgressive form of speech that violates her stance on the danger of words when she fears loss of Baines. Bluebeard's wife in the pageant within the film also uses a key to defy her husband and looks into a room of other wives' mutilated bodies. Ada's transgression of a prohibition, sending a love message on a key, leads to mutilation, a castration/death equivalent.

Not only might Ada fear the dangerous consequences of speaking, her elective muteness also withholds words of affection to inflict discomfort or punishment on others. Her father speaks of Ada's dark talent, her stubbornness, perhaps reflected in the resistant pony in the establishment shot, and to her potential for self-punitiveness. His belief that she can will herself to stop breathing foreshadows her nearly suicidal venture under water.

The abandonment theme is poignantly portrayed in Ada's symbolic delivery from the turbulent New Zealand sea when no one is there for her and Flora on the deserted beach. Her new husband also abandons her beloved piano and leaves her to buy land the day after she arrives. She feels enraged, helpless and powerless. But she can control whether she talks.

We witness Ada's silent anger after Stewart discovers her affair with Baines and imprisons her by boarding up the house. In her rage, she sadistically and manipulatively plays her husband at his core conflict. In order to gain her freedom she approaches Stewart as though to placate him and convince him that she has relinquished Baines and now desires her husband. But her ambiguous approach to this sexually awkward and passive man, called 'dry balls' by the Maori, humiliates and unmans him. She remains in full control by not allowing him to touch her. She repeatedly and manipulatively pulls down his garments even after he pulls them up with clenched fists. Instead of fondling his genitals her fingers stroke his buttocks and then slide down between his cheeks as though to penetrate him. Although aroused by this bewildering touch, he also appears besieged by a confusing mixture of humiliation, helplessness and anger. He cannot tolerate the equivalent of a homosexual penetration.

Later, when Flora gives Stewart the piano key with her mother's love message to Baines, Stewart's narcissistic rage at Ada's multiple deceptions leads him to retaliate by chopping off part of the finger that humiliated him and through which she 'talks' by signing and playing the piano. Furthermore, he identifies with both the aggressors: Ada who humiliated and symbolically castrated him, and Baines who tricked him in the land-for-piano barter and cuckolded him. He wields an axe like Bluebeard so that Ada, rather than he, is the castrated victim.

Ada uses her piano, touching and signing as substitutes for her voice. The piano is a poignant transitional object linked to the absence of her mother; Ada's playing, a wish for affectionate dialogue and touching with a pre-verbal mother. When deprived of her piano/ mother, Ada transforms a table into piano keys that she touches and seems to hear. Campion's camera lingers on Ada's touching with either side of her fingers almost everyone or everything in sight. She searches at the pre-verbal level for contact and solace.

When Ada commits herself to Baines, the need for her mother diminishes, and we see her struggle to relinquish her mother/piano. Ada tempts a suicidal death by placing her foot in the umbilical-like rope that pulls her down into the sea towards a permanent maternal connection. But in a symbolic rebirth or resurrection, Ada manages to free herself, attaining the developmental step of a commitment with a man.

The epilogue initially appears to be pure Hollywood. It is not. The metal fingertip ('I am quite the town freak') remains. Rather than allow all of her senses to be intact, she shrouds her head, her vision, in a black cloth as she attempts to speak. The film ends in an eerie and provocative dissolve. As Ada's piano rests on the sea bed, its lid fallen away, she floats above, her hair unbound, her arms stretched out in a gesture of surrender or crucifixion. Her body slowly turns on the end of the umbilical-like rope to the piano. The fronds of rust-coloured seaweed reach out to touch her like fibria as she remains fixed in her ambivalent connection to the womb.

In a voice-over at the end of the film:

At night I think of my piano in its ocean grave,
and sometimes of myself floating above it. Down
there everything is so still and silent that it
lulls me to sleep. It is a weird lullaby and so
it is; it is mine.

Is this silence the silence of her lost mother? Ada finds a caring husband but seems to continue her struggle with rage at abandonment, shame, depression and suicidal visions of suspension under the sea. Hovering over her lost piano/mother, she dreams of the imprisoning silence of death.

12. OVER-EXPOSURE:
TERRY ZWIGOFF'S *CRUMB*

ERIC J. NUETZEL, St. Louis

Documentary films complicate the task of psychoanalytic film criticism; they are renderings of fact, not fiction. They try not to traffic in the realm of fantasy, except as a subject, as they strive to disturb the viewer with difficult truths. Yet their aesthetic effect is under the influence of their film-maker's subjectivity. Conscious as well as unconscious identifications, transferences, countertransferences and resistances inevitably complicate the film-maker's interpretation of events, and shape the presentation.

Terry Zwigoff's *Crumb* seems no exception. The film is, by design, a psychobiography, a film portrait of the famed underground cartoonist and sketch artist R. (for Robert) Crumb. Robert burst into American consciousness in the late nineteen sixties with his hallucinogen inspired stream-of-consciousness cartoon style. With its own terrifying cuteness, Robert's art aims to skewer psychosocial and psychosexual hypocrisy. For better or for worse, his art is raw, honest and astonishingly revealing. In an interview after completion of the film, Zwigoff emphasised that he wanted to be as honest about Robert as Robert is in his own work, and added that if erred it was on the side of harshness (Sragow, 1995, pp. 13 & 20). A former psychology major and close friend of the artist, Zwigoff was in his own therapy as he exposed his famous friend on film. Zwigoff takes us into Robert's life, past as well as present, and into the heart of his deeply troubled family. His film is a disturbing meditation on creativity, trauma, character pathology, perversion, and the variability of psychopathology expressed in three brothers: Robert, his older brother Charles, and his younger brother Maxon. Two sisters would not participate. Robert found viewing the film 'excruciating' (Crumb & Crumb, 1995, p. 96).

Robert's provocatively misogynistic and racist cartoons are the subject of debate in Zwigoff's film. Are these cartoons scathing social satire or transgressive trash? The viewer is left to decide. Deirdre English, former editor of *Mother Jones*, observes that Robert's cartoon panels reveal the artist's insecurity, his sense of powerlessness relating to women. In contrast, art critic Robert Hughes compares him to Bruegel and Goya. Journalist Peggy Orenstein reports how much Robert's depictions of women and sex disturbed her in her adolescence. Fellow cartoonists and former publishers, male and female, celebrate or condemn Robert's provocative work. Zwigoff introduces us to Robert's art through carefully constructed montage sequences. There are revealing interviews with the artist and all those who surround him. Zwigoff, through Robert, reminds us of Sigmund Freud's aphorism by showing us Robert's sketch of an aggressive female nude with the caption 'Anatomy is destiny', as the nude invites the viewer to 'Check it out, sucker'. Later, Dian Hanson, a female pornographer and Robert's former lover, observes that men who prefer breasts are athletic and outgoing, while men who prefer legs are anxious and insecure—seeking a powerful mommy. She teases Robert as the latter type, only later to rhapsodise about his large

penis. Zwigoff's presentation expresses his admiration for the artist, and offers a wild formulation relating to Robert's singular success.

Robert's cartoon images include buxom women with heads of
protruding sharp-beaked predatory birds; naked men diving into
an oversized, ample woman from the rear; an African-American
woman being tricked by a group of white men who dunk her head
into a toilet; a bearded character, Mr Natural, lending his headless
girlfriend to a friend for sex, and so on. In Robert's depictions of
sexual intercourse, the man always enters the woman from
behind. The female buttocks appear large, and the vulva appears
meaty. Many of the women appear to be androgynous. White male
authority is abusive or corrupt, priapic boys are giddy, weak men
are nervous wrecks, and women are stupid, headless, and/or allur-
ing phallic-androgynous she-devils. In the film, Robert tells us
that he masturbates to his sexually explicit renderings of the
female form. His sexuality emerged in childhood through an
erotic fixation on Bugs Bunny. Later, he developed a shoe/boot
fetish. Currently his preferred form of sexual foreplay is a piggy-
back ride. Zwigoff's presentation suggests that castration anxiety
has structured a regression to an insecure, fetishistic, and ambivalent phallic-narcissism. Robert disdains male power, as he revels
in it. Although he sometimes wants to take her head off, the familiar fantasy of the phallic woman seems to appeal to him as an
unburdening solution. Dian Hanson (above) may have a point.

The experiential past that informs Robert's perversely enter-
taining style is clarified by the film-maker's inquisitive camera.
When we first meet the artist we observe him free associating

with his pen, as he tells of drawing to keep from being suicidal; although sometimes he feels suicidal as he draws. The first picture we see him working on is of himself, oppressed by a large camera, appearing ill with the caption, 'I'm nauseous'. The image is shown to us again near to the end of the film with this quote above the image and caption; 'How perfectly goddamned delightful it all is, to be sure', attributed to his older brother, Charles. Robert has every reason to feel queasy. The film demonstrates that his unsettling themes and idiosyncratic predilections contain the residue of a seriously disturbed early family life. What emerges is a portrait of creativity as partial sublimation; here artistic talent serves as a container for drives shaped by overstimulation and abuse. His two brothers did not fare as well.

The three brothers share a deeply traumatic past, all three have artistic talent; yet one is a world famous cartoonist, another a suicide, and another subsists marginally. Why? The film underscores the role of the family environment, constitution notwithstanding. Their father, an ex-marine and corporate businessman, abused his children physically, breaking Robert's collar bone when the artist was 5 years old. The eldest child, Charles, bore the brunt of father's sadism. Zwigoff's film tells us that father, now deceased, wrote a book entitled *Training People Effectively*, and that mother became an amphetamine addict when Robert was 9 years old.

She would attack father and scratch his face until it bled. She gave her children enemas. In childhood, Charles, Robert, and their younger siblings Maxon and two sisters formed the Animaltown Publishing Company. Charles had become obsessed with drawing cartoons, and forced his younger siblings to draw with him. On film Maxon says the brothers were 'three primordial monkeys working it out in the trees'. We are left to wonder what else went on.

Maxon, who appears schizophreniform, reveals to Zwigoff's camera that he now suffers with epilepsy, has a history of impulsive sexual assaults on unsuspecting women, meditates on a bed of nails, and periodically purifies his intestines by swallowing a thin length of cloth that eventually passes through his system. Charles, plagued by masochism, psychosis, and depression committed suicide within the year after Zwigoff filmed him. Robert appears cynical, depressive, and reclusive. His artistic success has enabled him to transcend self-destructiveness and eccentric isolation. In his cartoon world, Robert can be safely outrageous. His celebrity draws others to him, especially women. His second wife and fellow cartoonist, Aline, tolerates his proclivities.

The film takes place as Robert and Aline prepare to move to the South of France (her idea) with their daughter. In the film, as the moving van arrives, Robert denies any attachment to Charles, who taught him to draw. He says of leaving Charles, 'What do I care?' A few frames later Zwigoff undermines Robert's denial. For Robert, emotional detachment promotes survival. Earlier in the film there are interviews with Charles, who, despite his ravaged life comes across as witty, soulful, intelligent and charming. His honest self-appraisal is heroic, and contrasts nicely with Robert's defensive disingenuousness. The gut-wrenching effect of Charles's suicide, announced in a bleak sentence as one of the final frames, punctuates the fact that Charles did matter, at least to Zwigoff. He dedicates the film, 'For Charles'.

The dedication angered me. I thought that Zwigoff was disin-
genuous, having exploited Charles to get Robert's story. Robert
and Aline were also disturbed by the film; they felt used by Zwigoff and depicted themselves in a cartoon as his marionettes
(Crumb & Crumb, 1995).

Other viewers have told me of feeling guilty about Charles's suicide, as if their voyeurism colluded in his demise. This effect may be
exactly what Zwigoff was after; it may be close to what he felt. Zwigoff presents himself as transgressive; he elicits these responses. In an
early film sequence, he shows Robert on the telephone talking to
someone (presumably Robert's mother), as Robert is told that
Charles doesn't want to be filmed. Then he and Robert are in
Charles's room filming Charles anyway. Did they obtain consent?
Does a film-maker have an obligation to do no harm? Zwigoff may
give us his take through his construction of the film; the edited interviews with Charles seem to have been selected for hints of what was
to come. Could this lead to the impression, in some viewers, that the
film and its events may have contributed to Charles's suicide? Is
this effect unintentional or intentional? Regardless, Zwigoff's construction seems harsh with himself, and with Robert. The motives for
Charles's suicide were buried with him, but undoubtedly they were
more complex than the film could possibly expose. I suspect that
Zwigoff knows this. His portrait of Robert and the family Crumb
does demonstrate that comedy intermingles with tragedy, artistic
creativity wrestles with subjectively experienced trauma, psychosis
amplifies self-destructiveness, fetishism refracts phallocentric conflict, and although psychological detachment may be adaptive at
times, it can be overdone. The film is a remarkable document.

REFERENCES

CRUMB, R. & CRUMB, C. (1995). 'Head for the hills! Trying to escape the "R. Crumb Thing"'. *The New Yorker Magazine*, 24 April, pp. 96-7

SRAGOW, M. (1995). The man behind the man in *Crumb*. *The New York Times*, 23 April, Section H.

13. NARRATING DESIRE AND DESIRING NARRATION: A PSYCHOANALYTIC READING OF *THE ENGLISH PATIENT*

DIANA DIAMOND, NEW YORK

The English Patient plunges the viewer into an ambiguous world of visual splendour: a wash of luminous golden colour, a brush drawing a figure on a grainy surface, a hieroglyphic, a swimmer, a woman swimmer; contours suggestive of the desert or a woman's body. The figure floats over desert dunes, until it merges with the shadow of a small plane carrying a woman, pale and seemingly asleep, and a man, a pilot with goggles and a leather helmet. As the plane flies over a desert ridge, it is fired upon by German troops. The figures become incandescent with fire, and as the man falls burning from the sky, 'the flames erase all that matters—his name, his past, his face, his lover' (Minghella et al., 1996, p. 4).

In subsequent scenes the figures first seen soaring over the desert are replaced by the image of a man lying in the sand burned beyond recognition. We hear his laboured breathing, we view the Bedouin caravan, the itinerant Arab doctor, the searing sun in part through his makeshift mask of plaited palm leaves; and these shots of perceptual subjectivity establish our primary filmic identification with this anonymous man who comes to be called simply, 'the English Patient'. Among the few possessions that survive the smoking wreckage of the plane is a worn leather-bound volume of the *Histories* by Herodotus, filled with letters and clippings, in which is a drawing of the film's opening image of the female figure.

These two artifacts, the figure drawing and Herodotus's *Histories*, introduce the film's major theme—the centrality of representation and narrative, both imagistic and lexical, to human experience. It is not until later in the film that we learn that the constructed figure, the first image of the film, is a replica of human figure paintings in the cave of swimmers; figures that were copied by an Englishwoman Katherine Clifton and given to the Hungarian Count Laszlo De Almasy, an explorer and discoverer of the cave paintings, to paste in his copy of the *Histories* as a remembrance of their time in the desert, and as an emblem of their as yet unspoken, but palpable love for each other. The opening image of the swimming figure thus foretells the film's personal narrative—the reconstruction of the identity of Almasy (the English patient)—and the film's historical narrative—the exploration of the desert by the Royal Geographic Society of which Almasy was a member, and its colonisation during World War II.

This review interprets *The English Patient* in the light of controversies about the nature and construction of narrative in contemporary analytic theory and practice—the interconnection between narrative and identity (Ricoeur, 1985; Schafer, 1992); the relevance of relationships, both transferential and otherwise to narrative construction (Hanly, 1996); and the points of contact and divergence between narrative and historical truth (Schafer, 1982, 1992; Spence, 1982). My use of clinical psychoanalytic theory towards an analysis of a cinematic text is inspired by the potential interplay between psychoanalytic narrative processes

and cinematic narratives, and their impact on the spectator (Gabbard, 1997; Hanly, 1996).

The English Patient is about the reconstruction of Almasy's identity and life history, an account in which historical and narrative
truth increasingly converge as he engages more and more deeply
with significant objects in his life, both internal and external. Identity is constructed in part through the accounts that we give about
ourselves and our lives (Ricoeur, 1985), and these accounts often
comprise a set of varied narratives which reflect varied selves
(Schafer, 1992). *The English Patient* constantly reworks the story of
Almasy's life in flashbacks that initially have the idiosyncratic and
poetic-disjunctive quality of free associations, but that later cohere
into a chronological account of his life that he recreates for himself
and others.

In this zigzag movement from the private world of memory and
desire to the creation of a shared consensual account, the narrative
configurations of *The English Patient* to a certain extent parallel the
process of narrative construction in analysis. The assumption of the
anonymous identity of the English patient represents a screen narrative (Kris, 1956) which incorporates aspects of the identities of
lost others. A man burned beyond recognition lies in a convalescent
hospital in Italy, capable of giving only the most truncated and fragmented account of his life to the British officer who questions him
and to Hana, the French-Canadian nurse who cares for him. Indeed,
Almasy first depicts himself as Geoffrey Clifton, Katherine's husband, a British undercover agent, and recollects images related to
him by Katherine, whose memories of her garden sloping down to
the sea figured in her last words to Almasy as she lay dying in the

cave of swimmers. It is not so much that the English patient has forgotten his name and identity, as that he is resistant to knowing it, as is the case with many analysands.

This screen identity also serves to protect the English patient from the falsifying narratives imposed upon him by others. The English patient is a man whose personal narrative and self-definition as an internationalist opposed to colonisation and ownership, are at variance with the official narratives that circulated during World War II—narratives which affirmed nationalism, borders and ownership. Reflecting on the deforming aspects of such official narratives, Maddox, Almasy's close friend and colleague in the Royal Geographic Society, states, 'It's ghastly, like a witch hunt—anybody remotely foreign is suddenly a spy ... We didn't care about countries ... Brits, Arabs, Hungarians, Germans. None of that mattered ... It was something finer than that' (Minghella et al., 1996, p. 148).

Like the analyst in the consulting room, the spectator of *The English Patient* must penetrate the screen of the patient's obfuscating and partial narratives to construct the patient's identity and history on the basis of his associations and memories, and the viewer's own corresponding associations, inferences and internal schemata (Bordwell, 1985). The complexities of the film's narrative discourse, including the rapid shifts between scenes in Egypt and Italy, between intertwined narratives of the English patient and his nurse Hana, between past and present, visual and verbal narrative mechanisms, places the spectator at the heart of narrative construction.

The dislocations of regular chronology, point of view, and spatial and temporal conventions in *The English Patient* redouble the tasks of the spectator because they create a disjunction between the storyline or fabula (e.g. the chronological order of events with their spatial, temporal and causal dimensions) and the sjuzet (e.g. the order of events as it is depicted in narrative discourse, or in the actual unfolding of scenes, actions, turning points in the text) (Bordwell, 1985; Brooks, 1984). Such disjunctions, often conveyed in film through flashbacks as is the case in *The English Patient*, are meant to impede as well as advance the spectator's understanding. The tension between fabula and sjuzet thus demands that the spectator not only constantly recode the film's imagery into a set chronology, but also like an analyst comprehend and construct the nature of characters' inner experience that leads to such narrative fractures and delays.

The English Patient reflects aspects of analytic process not only in its demand on the spectator and in its cinematic techniques which mirror free association, but also in its emphasis on the creation of a shared narrative, shaped not only by the patient's images, words and affects, but also by their affective resonance in Hana. It is the patient's relationship with Hana, the French-Canadian nurse who retreats with him to the abandoned Italian monastery of St Anna de Prenzi that enables Almasy to turn his attention and interest once again to his inner experiences and memories. Schafer (1982, 1992) has reconceptualised free association in the light of narrative theory as fragments of life stories created as they are related in the context of the analytic relationship. Just as the patient in analysis tells his or her own story to the analyst, who listens and tries to make sense of it, so does Hana immerse herself in reconstructing the English patient's narrative, searching for coherence and continuity in its chaotic configurations, and bridging its chasms and lacunae.

Hana's willingness to become the co-explorer of the English patient's psychic space simultaneously reawakens his desire and fuels his desire for narration. The reawakening of desire and its connection with narrative creation is depicted cinematically through a series of flashbacks that merge past and present. As Hana reads the story of Candaulles and his Queen from the patient's worn memento-filled copy of the *Histories* by Herodotus, the camera pans to reveal a spellbound Almasy gazing on Katherine telling the same story, her being illuminated by the fire from the camp of the Royal Geographic Society. Just as Candaulles urges his friend Gyres to gaze on his naked Queen in the original and timeless sphere of the myth that Hana reads to the patient from Herodotus' *Histories*, so does the English patient gaze on Hana in the present, and finally and most vividly, in memory, on Katherine as she dramatises the story in the past.

The use of the filmic technique of cross-cutting from present to past, as though the past were located in space rather than time, establishes the simultaneity of past and present as veridical regions. This cinematic condensation of space and time establishes the present and past as coexisting sheets or strata in the psyche 'each region with its own characteristics, its "tones", its "aspects", its "singularities", its "shining points" and its "dominant themes"' (Deleuze, 1989, p. 99). The specific tones of past and present are enhanced by the cinematic depiction of the past world (e.g. the world of the desert) in bright bold tones and clear crisp images. In contrast, the present world (e.g. the world of the monastery of St

Anna De Prenzi) is depicted in a series of diffuse, muted watery tones and long liquidy shots (Minghella et al., 1996), which render the present dreamlike and indistinct. This juxtaposition of vivid past with muted present reverses the usual pattern of films with two time scales and brings a sense of urgency, immediacy and heightened reality to the past.

The parallels between the English patient and his nurse, and that of an analyst and analysand are, of course, limited. As Gabbard (1997) points out, we cannot talk about a psychoanalytic process without the patient's associations and the here-and-now lively interplay of transference and countertransference, free association and resistence. However, echoes of such elements do appear in the film. The complex relationship between Hana and the patient is transferential in nature for both, in that they each represent a new object for the other, which is identified with past objects. However, just as in an analysis, this new object relationship revives old unconscious wishes, fears and conflicts, which catalyse new development, but also create new distortions. For example, the patient's recollections of his relationship with Katherine are motivated not only by his need to reconstruct his story and identity, but also by his need to again be known and fully seen by another (Hana). However, the patient presents only kaleidoscopic fragments of his past, fragments which captivate Hana, but which obscure the more ambiguous and problematic aspects of his history and identity. In a similar vein, Hana sees the patient through the distorting mirror of her own wartime losses of fiancé, father and best friend. After the latter is killed in a land-mine explosion, Hana asks the patient, 'I must be a curse ... anyone who loves me, anyone who gets close to me, or I must be cursed. Which is it?' Her participation in the creation of the patient's identity is clearly reparative in nature; but it also functions to help her evade painful aspects of her own identity and experience. Thus, the transference love between the patient and Hana—as in an analysis—both facilitates understanding and transformation, and becomes a source of resistance and avoidance.

Just as the English patient recovers the depth of his passion for Katherine through Hana's ministrations to him, both physical and psychological, so does Hana come emotionally alive again through her association with the sensuous, enigmatic Kip, a Sikh member of the British army who takes up residence in their region to defuse land mines. A complete discussion of Hana's relationship to Kip and its parallels to Almasy's relationship to Katherine is beyond the scope of this paper. However, both relationships illustrate how passion may catalyse human symbolic expression, as well as the forces of potential destruction. Indeed, Kip's dangerous specialty of land-mine sweeping itself may represent the excavation of libidinal and aggressive forces, eros and thanatos that forms part of any analytic process.

The convergence between the two relationships is reinforced in the magical scene where Kip shows Hana the spectacular frescoes by Piero della Francesca in a Tuscan church by candlelight, a scene which parallels Almasy's discovery of the cave of swimmers, and its revelation to Katherine, earlier in the film. Both scenes, which involve the illumination of images in the context of darkness, are also a metaphor for the visual pleasures that cinema affords us. As Hana swings through space, the rope encircling her waist manipulated by Kip who is in darkness, illuminating the frescoes with her flare, giving us glimpses of faces, bodies and angels, we are reminded how much visualisation, like representation, emerges from a relational context. Hana's exhilaration, rapture and kinesthetic movements are reminiscent both of erotic desire (Minghella et al., 1996) and of early rocking and holding. The array of luminous but fleeting cinematic images re-evokes the process of the early visualisation that emerges erratically out of the matrix of early mother–child transactions, where the mother's face and form become the vehicle for visual construction, just as Kip becomes the vehicle for Hana's visual pleasure (Lichtenberg, 1983; Diamond & Wrye, 1998).

The two film clips just shown indicate that desire, as it is scenarised in *The English Patient* is depicted to have both oedipal and pre-oedipal roots, both of which infuse the film's narrative mechanisms. Part of the film's ubiquitous appeal is undoubtedly the triangular relationship between Almasy, Katherine and her husband Geoffrey (and the corresponding triangle between Hana, Kip and the patient), with its timeless oedipal themes of desire and renunciation, rivalry and pursuit, betrayal and loss that often characterise classic Hollywood narrative films (Gabbard & Gabbard, 1990). As Barthes states, 'Today we dismiss Oedipus and narrative as one and the same; we no longer love, we no longer fear, we no longer narrate' (1975, p. 47). But the intense admixture of love and aggression, misogyny and obsession, raw sexuality and tenderness, possessiveness and repudiation that characterises Almasy's love for Katherine clearly contains preoedipal as well as oedipal derivatives, as do most love relationships (Kernberg, 1995). Significantly, after he makes love to Katherine, Almasy plays the Hungarian folk song 'Szerelem, Szerelem' (love, love) which he tells her was sung to him by his Daijka (nurse) when he was a child in

Budapest. Heard episodically from the opening takes of the film, this plaintive folk song functions as an 'acoustic mirror' (Silverman, 1988), a vocal evocation of Almasy's early sensuous preverbal experience, and its significance for his dual interlinked passions for exploring Katherine's body and the desert. Indeed, we first see Almasy in dialogue with an ancient Arab, drawing a map of a ridge that is likened to the curve of a woman's back. Later in the film, contemplating the hollow at the base of Katherine's throat, Almasy states: 'I love this place, what's it called—this is mine ... I'm going to ask the king permission to call it the Almasy Bosphorous' (Minghella et al., 1996, pp. 100–101).

In his exploration of both Katherine's body and the desert we see echoes of Klein's observation that the imperative to explore is often a derivative of early 'phantasies of exploring the mother's body' (1975, p. 333). The admixture of aggression, love, curiosity and greed in such early phantasies, as well as the impossibility of realising them, leads the child to substitute a territory for mother, a territory in which he can escape, recreate and realise the early attachment. The thrust towards exploration is also bound up with the desire for reparation; that is, with the desire to restore and replenish the good things that the child phantasises he/she has plundered from the mother's body—a body which Klein reminds us is often unconsciously equated with the earth.

In *The English Patient* Katherine is equated with the dangerous, treacherous land (motherland) that must not only be explored, but subdued and conquered. At the same time, Katherine represents a genre of women travellers and explorers in film who, as Kaplan (1997) observes, accentuate their feminine masquerade to avoid reprisal for their strivings. Such women, with their combination of strength and vulnerability, pose a challenge to the often tenuous sense of masculinity of the men around them, who also are prey to terrors of the unknown. These fears are often projected, as in the scene where Almasy cautions Clifton not to leave his wife in the desert because it is too harsh. Clifton's reply, 'Why are you all so afraid of a woman?' speaks to the projected anxieties described above. Hence we must see Almasy's gaze on Katherine as not only a subjective and adoring one that seeks mutual recognition, but as an objectifying one that seeks domination and control over its object (Kaplan, 1997).

Such an objectifying, dominating gaze subtly distorts the perception of Arabs as well as women in the film. The Palestinian poet Hussein Barghouti sums up the portrayal of Arabs in *The English Patient* as follows: 'Foreground action: white people, noble fine feelings, strong full of laughter, walking in gardens, taking showers, standing up. Background action: Arabs, shifty, mysterious, dirty, untrustworthy, sitting down' (quoted in Hare, 1998, p. 34). Such a view is discrepant with the conscious ideology of the film contained in Maddox's nostalgic rendering of the camaraderie of the Royal Geographic Society cited earlier: 'We didn't care about countries ... Brits, Arabs, Hungarians, Germans. None of that mattered ... It was something finer than that' (Minghella et al., 1996, p. 148). Such discrepancies between verbal and visual, lexical and imagistic filmic texts remind us that *The English Patient*, like most commercial Hollywood films, is structured through an interplay of contradictory and diverse codes, which together convey the film's conscious and unconscious ideology about gender and nationality. The film text may thus be said to be fissured; evidence of such fissures is found in such contradictions between lexical and imagistic depictions and in breaks in narration.

An example of such a narrative fissure is the account that Almasy gives to Katherine about the song 'Szerelem, Szerelem'. He tells Katherine that this lullaby that was sung to him by his Hungarian nurse is really 'the story of a Hungarian count, he's a wanderer, a fool. For years he's on some kind of quest, for—who knows what? And then one day he falls under the spell of a mysterious English woman—a Harpy—who beats him and hits him and he becomes her slave and sews her clothes and worships the hem of her' (Minghella et al., 1996, p. 100).

This fantasy reveals that, for Almasy, intimacy with Katherine unearths primitive anxieties about subjugation to an all-powerful female object, as evidenced by the gender role reversal implied in Almasy's fantasy quoted above (Person, 1985; Stoller & Herdt, 1982; Wrye, & Welles, 1982, 1994).

Indeed, the relationship between Katherine and Almasy capsizes in the maelstrom of such primitive anxieties; for them, reparative strivings come too late. In contrast, the relationship between Hana and Almasy offers the possibility for the expression of reparative strivings for both, which in turn enables them each to fully reconstitute their lost objects in memory. 'Why are you so determined to keep me alive?' asks the patient. Hana's deceptively simple reply, 'Because I am a nurse', evokes such reparative themes. One also senses that the patient stays alive because he senses that Hana needs him to do so, and thus his repeated statements to her, 'I'm still here' (Minghella et al., 1996, p. 64).

If the relationship between Hana and the English patient epitomises the reparative nature of narrative insights that emerge from a here-and-now telling to another, other aspects of the film remind us that such narrative constructions may be partial. Reconstruction of historical aspects of patients' lives, with reference to early life circumstances is essential for the development of a complete and comprehensive narrative (Hanly, 1996). One such source of past history is the Herodotus itself, written, as the English patient tells Katherine, by the father of history. The volume of the Herodotus, which merges mythic, personal and historical narratives, provides clues to the patient's ambiguous identity and history, and catalyses the multiple flashbacks which are the film's primary narrative mechanism. As such, it embodies the film's reverence for narration, its centrality to Almasy's past as well as present life, but also affirms the importance of historical reconstruction, or of locating narrative in the context of history, individual, social and political. Almasy first affirms the depth of his emotional connection to Katherine when he agrees to paste her copies of the cave paintings into his book. She in turn becomes aware of his love for her when she sees her name in the *Histories* where Katherine also records her final words, as she lies dying in the cave of swimmers, waiting for Almasy to return.

The *Histories* by Herodotus also becomes the vehicle for the recognition of Almasy by Caravaggio, the Canadian spy who has been tortured and mutilated by the Germans—as an inadvertent result of Almasy's actions during war. 'I saw you writing in that book. At the embassy in Cairo when I had thumbs and you had a face and a name', he tells Almasy (Minghella et al., 1996, p.52). Initially, Caravaggio is also a vehicle for the introduction of the type of distorted narrative that can be created when the actualities or consequences of one's actions are separated from their subjective meaning or intent. As such, his presence is depicted as sinister and menacing, like the crows that Hana chases from her garden in the scene just before Caravaggio appears at the monastery gate.

Caravaggio poses a challenge to the shared narrative forged by Hana and Almasy, suggesting that the English patient may not be English at all, but instead Hungarian and a Nazi collaborator. He introduces certain historical realities, some of them heretofore unknown to the patient and/or to Hana, without which Almasy's understanding of his life and fate would be incomplete. For example, Almasy learns from Caravaggio that Maddox, his best friend and colleague in the Royal Geographic Society, shot himself when he learned that Almasy had given their expedition maps, which showed the way through the desert, to the Germans in exchange for a plane that would enable him to return to the injured Katherine. Confronted for the first time with the full historical, as well as personal, ramifications of his love for Katherine, Almasy recreates for Caravaggio the full circumstances of his betrayal by and of the British, including his unjust incarceration as a Nazi collaborator and spy and his unwitting complicity in the deaths of both Katherine and Geoffrey Clifton. 'So yes she died because of me, because I loved her, because I had the wrong name' (Minghella et al., 1996, p. 166).

By integrating historical actualities, derived from confrontations with Caravaggio and with his own writings in the *Histories,* and subjective realities, derived from his mutual exchanges with Hana, Almasy finally becomes the agent in the creation of his own narrative (Schafer, 1996). The multiple versions, images and points of view are woven into a complex tapestry of his own design, making Almasy, 'one person telling stories about single selves, multiple selves, fragments of selves and selves of different sorts ...' (Schafer, 1992, p. 51). The creation of such a monistic and integrative narrative, that blends narrative and historical truth, enables the patient finally to die, and Hana finally to relinquish him. (In one of the film's most poignant moments, he communicates his readiness for death nonverbally by silently pushing a lethal dose of morphine ampules towards Hana as she prepares his daily injection.) Just as narrative construction was at the centre of his life, so, too, does it ease his way into death. As he dies, Hana reads to him Katherine's last words, and the camera discloses Katherine on the eve of her death, writing in the *Histories* as she awaits Almasy's return to the cave of swimmers. 'We die, rich with lovers and tribes, tastes we have swallowed ... bodies we have entered and swum up like rivers, fears we have hidden in like this wretched cave ... I want all this marked on my body. We are the real countries, not the boundaries drawn on maps with the name of powerful men ... that's all I've ever wanted—to walk in such a place with you, with friends, an earth without maps' (Minghella et al., 1996, pp. 171–172).

As she reads, Hana's voice alternates with that of Katherine, until the two women, the two storylines, past and present, and the two types of representation, imagistic and lexical, visual and verbal, merge into one restorative narrative in which past experience is recovered, represented and mourned.

The English patient's death is rendered bearable because the narrative of his life has been completed and will endure, visualised

symbolically by Hana scooping up the *Histories* lying on the bedside
table as she leaves the monastery for the last time. In its final integration of past and present, memory and actuality, narrative and
historical truth, the film's concluding sequence cuts from Hana
catching a last glimpse of the monastery from the back of a truck
driven by Caravaggio, to a long shot of Almasy and Katherine in the
cockpit of a plane, clearing the ridge of the Gilf Kebir and the Cave
of Swimmers, and then soaring freely over the desert, this time its
contours fully defined and unmistakable.

Acknowledgements: The author gratefully acknowledges the contributions of Drs Emanuel Berman, Catherine Portuges and Harriet Wrye. This paper is dedicated to the memory of Madge
Friedman Alschuler in acxknowledgement of a life so gracefully
lived and so generously shared. Her account of her participation in
the Red Cross during World War II deepened my understanding of
the historical period depicted in this film.

REFERENCES

BARTHES, R. (1975). *The Pleasure of the Text*, trans. R. Miller. New
    York: Hill & Wang.
BORDWELL, D. (1985). *Narration in the Fiction Film*. Madison, WI:
    Univ. of Wisconsin Press.
BROOKS, P. (1984). *Reading for the Plot: Design and Intention in Nar-
    rative*. London and Cambridge, MA: Harvard Univ. Press.
DELEUZE, G. (1989). *Cinema 2*. Minneapolis: Univ. of Minnesota
    Press.

DIAMOND, D. & WRYE, H. (1998). Epilogue. Projections of psychic reality: a centennial of film and psychoanalysis. *Psychoanal. Inq.*, 18: 311–334.

GABBARD, G. O. (1997). The psychoanalyst at the movies. *Int. J. Psychoanal.*, 78, 429–434.

GABBARD, G. & GABBARD, K. (1990). Play it again, Sigmund. Psychoanalysis and the classic Hollywood text. *J. Popular Film & TV*, 18: 6–17.

HANLY, M. F. (1996). Narrative now and then: a critical realist approach. *Int. J. Psychoanal.*, 77: 445–457.

HARE, D. (1998). *Via Dolorosa & When Shall We Live?* London: Faber & Faber.

KAPLAN, E. A. (1997). *Looking for the Other: Feminism, Film and the Imperial Gaze.* New York and London: Routledge.

KERNBERG, O. (1995). *Love Relations.* New Haven and London: Yale Univ. Press.

KLEIN, M. (1975). *Love, Guilt, Reparation and Other Works. 1921–1945.* New York: Delta.

KRIS, E. (1956). The recovery of childhood memories in psychoanalysis. *Psychoanal. Study Child*, 11: 54–58.

LICHTENBERG, J. (1983). *Psychoanalysis and Infant Research.* Hillsdale, NJ: The Analytic Press.

MINGHELLA, A. ET AL. (1996). *The English Patient.* New York: Hyperion/ Miramax.

PERSON, E. (1985). The erotic transference in women and men: differences and consequences. *J. Amer. Acad. Psychoanal.*, 13: 159–80.

RICOEUR, P. (1985). History as narrative and practice. *Philosophy Today,* p. 214.

SCHAFER, R. (1982). The relevance of the here and now transference interpretation to the reconstruction of early development. *Int. J. Psychoanal.,* 63: 77–82.

—— (1992). *Retelling a Life: Narration and Dialogue in Psychoanalysis.* New York: Basic Books.

SILVERMAN, K. (1988). *The Acoustic Mirror.* Bloomington and Indianapolis, IN: Indiana Univ. Press.

SPENCE, D. (1982). *Narrative Truth and Historical Truth.* New York: Norton.

STOLLER, R. J. & HERDT, G. H. (1982). The development of masculinity: a cross-cultural contribution. *J. Amer. Psychoanal. Assn,* 30: 29–59.

WRYE, H. K. & WELLES, J. (1994). *The Narration of Desire.* Hillsdale, NJ: Analytic Press.

14. *THE REMAINS OF THE DAY*[1]

MECHTHILD ZEUL, MADRID

Freud felt that it was only possible to develop cogent and definitive conclusions from the clinical material of a psychoanalytic treatment after termination. In a similar vein, only after I had watched James Ivory's *The Remains of the Day* (1993) several times and had the entire film text in front of my inner eye was I able to develop some tentative interpretive formulations about the film. My basic methodology for approaching this film lies in the assumption that there is an exchange between the film and its interpretive audience that manifests itself in a network of multiple identifications. Reflections on these identifications reveal a direct connection to psychoanalytic theory. A new text is created that is anchored in the concrete data of the film but no longer resides exclusively or directly in the film images. Instead, the new text grows out of the psychoanalytic interpretation brought to bear on the film.

There is a parallel situation in the narrative of the film itself. Closely integrated are the collaboration of Lord Darlington with the Nazi regime and the unhappy love story between the housekeeper, Ms Kenton, and the butler, Stevens. The film deftly sketches the interrelationship of these two threads of action through a psychological portrait of the protagonist Stevens and his authoritarian, contemptuous behaviour towards others. In essence,

---

[1] Translated by Dean C. Collins.

The Remains of the Day is a social criticism film that depicts psycho-pathological preconditions for the socially recognised behaviour of an English butler. He is neutral towards the political convictions and moral values of his master—knowledge of them would greatly impede the fulfilment of his purpose in life, which is to serve loyally and unobtrusively. His one and only task is to carry out his master's orders and wishes in exquisite detail and without any reservations whatsoever.

Being of service has an inherent value for Stevens. The film persuasively depicts him as completely out of touch with his own feelings and thoughts, suggesting that in serving his master, he loses contact with himself. The object master has displaced his ego ideal. The tragedy of the film, though, is that through the willing internalisation of this object into his ego, he then depends on its physical and psychic presence to sustain meaning in his life or even life itself. Without explicitly stating this conclusion, the film certainly allows for an interpretive understanding that blind obedience to one's master through the internalisation of the honoured and valued object may lead to a transcendent form of narcissistic fulfilment. The master then completes the self in the sense of Kohut's description of the selfobject. As the film unfolds, the audience gradually reaches the chilling conclusion that internalisation and blind obedience of this nature may have been essential prerequisites for the amoral behaviour of the Germans that made possible the genocide of the Jews.

Hanns Sachs (1929, 'Zur Psychologie des Films' [On the psychology of the film]. *Die Psychoanalytische Bewegung*, I: 122–6), an early contributor to the psychoanalytic understanding of film, made the point that the medium of film can depict inner psychic connections only through externally perceptible events. A similar principle is applicable to *The Remains of the Day*. The death of his Lord Darlington leads Stevens to take a journey in his former master's car to the west coast of England, where he hopes to meet Ms Kenton after more than twenty years. This journey illustrates Stevens's internal conflict that operates outside his conscious awareness, namely that he is struggling with two forms of love, an object-centred love for Ms Kenton and a narcissistic love for his master. A critical inner reckoning centred on this conflict might have been possible if Stevens's ego was not totally absorbed in his narcissistic love for Lord Darlington. This absorption places him in a position where he is even less capable of loving another person than before the loss of his master. Even though the image of his master is only a regrettable caricature, this object has become a part of Stevens to the point where it provides him with the only self-esteem and self-worth that he has known. Ms Kenton's efforts to woo Stevens represent a serious threat to his life design and his self-worth.

The intoxicating devotion to his master and his beloved dependence on him made it possible for Stevens to participate in the magnificent conferences organised by Lord Darlington on his estate, apparently in the service of peace in Europe, but actually in collaboration with the Nazis. That he is a prisoner of his narcissistic love is poignantly depicted when Stevens's father dies. Rather than linger at the deathbed of his father, his unswerving loyalty to Lord Darlington leads him to listen to the vulgar singing of a blonde-braided Nazi diva. Moreover, Stevens's devotion to his master makes him blind to feelings of love and pity that Ms Kenton asks

him to share. When she implores him to prevent her marriage to
Mr Benn, which she is contemplating out of a sense of disappointment, Stevens is so identified with his master that he contemptu-
ously responds with suggestions regarding her work.

As the audience undergoes various identifications with Stevens,
Ms Kenton and other characters in the film, there is a dawning
recognition that Stevens takes masochistic pleasure in uncondi-
tional surrender to his master. Viewed from this perspective, the
journey to the west coast of England represents a last desperate
attempt to recapture the lost object to which Stevens is simultaneously masochistically bound. The sado-masochistic tie forestalls a
threatening depressive breakdown. Stevens's ambivalence about
reuniting with Ms Kenton is skilfully manifested in a pivotal
sequence when Stevens, driving his car, turns away from the
observer. Rather than ending up on the west coast with Ms
Kenton, he arrives in the square in front of Darlington Hall, where
the auction of his deceased master's estate is under way. The death
of this narcissistically valued object activates the repressed conflict between his devotion to his master and his growing love for
Ms Kenton. His interest in Ms Kenton has already been apparent
from his voyeuristic spying on her, although in that role his position as an observer guarantees him the necessary distance from
his love object.

The audience ultimately resigns itself to the fact that Stevens's
wish to defer masochistically to his master in order to be ruled is
stronger than his longing to enter into a love relationship with Ms
Kenton. Hence Stevens's trip ends within the walls of Darlington
Hall. The threat of dissolution of the self or depressive breakdown

associated with his love for Ms Kenton is so powerful that he must renounce his love for her. Stevens's masochistic pleasure in merger reappears in the final frame when the camera lets Darlington Hall slowly disappear in the green meadows and forests, leaving the audience with bitter-sweet feelings of yearning and renunciation.

15. DECONSTRUCTING *DIRTY HARRY*: CLINT EASTWOOD'S UNDOING OF THE HOLLYWOOD MYTH OF SCREEN MASCULINITY IN *PLAY 'MISTY' FOR ME*

RONALD BAKER, LONDON

Clint Eastwood attained super-star box office status as 'The Man with No Name' through Sergio Leone's *spaghetti westerns* in the nineteen sixties and Don Siegel films, especially *Dirty Harry* (1971), in which he played the title part. Eastwood exemplified the proto-typical macho male Hollywood hero: cold, refractory, cruel, sadistic, murderous, ferocious and seemingly invulnerable, his callous contempt and abuse extending no less to women than to men. However, in his directorial debut, *Play Misty For Me* (1971), Eastwood cast himself as a character whose vulnerability contrasted markedly with his iconic screen persona, a portrayal that anticipated themes that recurred ever more poignantly in his subsequent films.

In *Misty*, Eastwood plays an all-night disc jockey Dave Garver, a philanderer who has jeopardised his relationship with a girlfriend, Tobie (Donna Mills). They have temporarily parted but it is evident that he wishes to rebuild that relationship. A girl regularly requests Erroll Garner's ballad 'Misty', which he occasionally plays. One night Dave is picked up by Evelyn (Jessica Walter), the girl who likes 'Misty', in a bar. They agree to a one-night-stand with 'no strings'. Evelyn turns out to be a morbidly jealous and murderous psychotic. She invades Dave's life with ever-increasing intimidation and violence, including verbal abuse, stalking and humiliation in public. Later she slashes her wrists, tears his house apart, attacks him with a knife, severely injures his maid and murders a policeman investigating the case. When Evelyn is caught and imprisoned, Dave and Tobie negotiate a brief reconciliation. However, Evelyn is unexpectedly released and the terror resumes. She moves in with Tobie (who has not met her previously) as a room-mate, ties her up, threatens to murder her and stabs Dave when he tries to rescue her. A struggle ensues, Dave punches her over a balcony and she falls to her death. In the final scene Dave, bleeding and shaken, leans dependently on Tobie as she helps him to the car.

On first reading the script, Eastwood recalled an incident when he was about 20 when an older woman became obsessed with him, threatening suicide when he tried to end the liaison. He took an option on it and sought to film it, offering to appear in and direct it. The studio refused. One can infer that his wish to display vulnerability in the starring role may have concerned the studio, who may have feared that he would undermine his screen persona and lose his box-office appeal.

His performance took him from his established role of arch male chauvinist and secure representative of male supremacy, to that of a helpless, confused, anguished, distraught and phallically endangered man, who, in contrast to earlier roles, is entrapped in a threatening and terrifying nightmare and unable to find a way out of the impasse. The deconstruction of the male supremacist image thus began under his own direction. In doing so he showed an awareness and understanding of his singular movie personality. *Misty* portrayed that deconstruction with purposeful efficiency. This shift in

Eastwood's screen persona has been the subject of study by film scholars. Positions are polarised; for instance Bingham (1994) emphasises Eastwood's progressive undermining of his early screen persona, whereas Smith (1993) is sceptical, seeing his attempt at undermining his image of male dominance as an unimpressive empty gesture. This essay is a contribution to that debate.

Douglas (1974) has described the young Eastwood as a shy youth and as an actor whose trademark is violence but who abhors violence in real life. Knight (1974) described him as gentle, soft-spoken and self-effacing and difficult to reconcile with the violent screen parts. Knee, however, is somewhat sceptical about these contradictions, concluding an article devoted to *Misty* somewhat cynically: 'We ... see Eastwood's ... effort as indicative of a *passing moment of progressive questioning* of traditional constructions of male identity prior to a conservative reaction which launched him into greater macho stardom' (1993, p. 101, my italics). He was, presumably, referring to Eastwood's next movie, *Dirty Harry* (1971).

In *Tightrope* (1984), directed by Richard Tuggle, Eastwood plays Wes Block, a cop investigating serial murders of prostitutes but close to breakdown following his divorce. He is guilt-ridden by his need to use prostitutes and asks himself how can he be so loving and protective towards his young daughters, yet be so perverse with prostitutes? The themes introduced in *Misty* continue to develop. The macho persona is weakened, with Block accepting responsibility for and in conflict with his baser actions. Moreover, he wants to be a husband and father with a family life. Holmlund (1986) notes that the power of the women's movement is avowed through Block's involvement with Beryl (Genevieve Bujold), a feminist who is cast as a strong and respected woman, Block's lover and a rape crisis therapist, who helps him to confront and reverse his hostility towards women and recognise his personal need for closeness and trust. Indeed, Eastwood consistently and decisively moves in the direction of empowering debased women, frequently the prostitutes and rape victims of his early films, a matter of no little interest to feminists.

These themes are further advanced in *Unforgiven* (1992). William Munny (Eastwood) was once a gunfighter. He not only killed bad guys, but women and children too. In a classic statement he says, 'I used to be a sinner, a drinker, a killer'. He now despises those characters who contributed to his earlier screen persona. He also pays tribute to his wife, who helped him to reform. He was strengthened and made virtuous by the influence of a good woman. He is now an ageing farmer devoted to maintaining his motherless family, but weakened and angered by his wife's death. Thus, when he hears of a $1,000 bounty on the heads of two cowboys who carved up a prostitute, he cannot resist. He goes on to again kill and sin just as he did before his wife saved him. In the end he is again redeemed and becomes a successful San Francisco merchant.

Eastwood purchased the novel of *The Bridges of Madison County* (1995), intending to direct and star in the film version, with predictably sceptical responses. How can the Hollywood macho icon of all time be making a romantic woman's film? However, it is essentially a serious and responsible examination of marital fidelity in the context of a transient love affair. The emotional climax of *Bridges* is mature, with Streep and Eastwood renouncing their love for each other. Streep leaves the man behind and emerges empowered, with strength, with dignity and with virtue, despite having passionately expressed her sexuality and erotism.

To study Eastwood, consideration of the audience is essential. In the Leone and *Dirty Harry* films, his representation of masculinity is replete with horrific imagery of women being disempowered and deflowered but also of men brutally destroying each other. Fantasies of power, mastery, omnipotence and control are spawned in spectators, who identify with these characteristics in a narcissistic way (Neale, 1993, pp. 10-11). This narcissistic identification attaches itself to screen portrayals of male dominance, which in Eastwood's case carries compelling imagery of both hero and villain, for males and females. The denigration of women suggests a narcissistic idealisation of phallic superiority over the dehumanised female and her devalued genitalia with obvious homosexual implications. The penis is regarded as all-powerful and, with relief, the fear of the female genitalia is denied. Again, the sado-masochistic brutality of man competing with and castrating fellow man excites the male spectator, who witnesses the inhumanity of this with passive voyeuristic approval, in the safety of the cinema.

The identification with the hero of Eastwood's later movies also has narcissistic implications but it is operating at the healthier end of the spectrum, where humanity, creativity and compassion in interpersonal relationships are paramount. The female genitalia and the goodness of woman are equally valued, inviting the male to recognise his longing for a heterosexual partner and family. A man is strengthened, not weakened, by this awareness, a matter Eastwood conveys unequivocally to his audience. Psychoanalysts know that many male patients are threatened by this and deeply resistant to acknowledging it. Presumably Eastwood's male audience are similarly inclined.

Beginning with *Misty*, Eastwood has resolutely sought to undermine both his *Might-in sexuality and violence-makes-right* persona and the narcissistic male spectator attracted to that image. Movies promise access to violence as an escape, but if that alone was on offer, it seems unlikely that Eastwood would retain his mass audience, who still include his pre-*Misty* fans. After all, it is the frustrations inherent in the moral demands of a repressive society that drive people to escapes such as those offered by the popular cinema. Violence continues to be present in most Eastwood films in sufficient quantity to satisfy primitive instincts. This may be a vital factor that continues to draw audiences, despite the underlying conflict-arousing message.

No previous actor/director has himself systematically deconstructed an iconic screen persona of such distinct and devastating male patriarchal tendency. Moreover, in the process Eastwood has addressed feminism, family values, responsibility of the individual, the roots of violence and the previously devalued strength that resides in a woman's dignity and virtue. He has methodically empowered women, but in addition he has confronted men in so far as he has forced them to rethink what it means to be masculine, through his courageous portrayal of himself in sharp contrast with his earlier screen image. The traditional Hollywood myth of masculinity is thus challenged and undone by the icon of screen patriarchy himself. Psychoanalysts may have neglected Eastwood's movies because the violence is perceived as being the same as that in the pre-*Misty* era. Women too have found it difficult to recognise the post-macho Eastwood, despite his explicit commitment to women's rights, again because of the overarching violence that continues to foster his image as a man's man. This brief essay may prompt a reappraisal.

REFERENCES

BINGHAM, D. (1994). *Acting Male: Masculinities in the Films of James Stewart, Jack Nicholson and Clint Eastwood*. New Brunswick, NJ: Rutgers Univ. Press.

DOUGLAS, P. (1974). *Clint Eastwood: Movin' On*. Chicago, IL: Henry Regnery.

HOLMLUND, C. (1986). Sexuality and power in the male doppelganger cinema: the case of Clint Eastwood's *Tightrope*. *Cinema J.*, 26: 31-42.

KNEE, A. (1993). The dialectic of female power and male hysteria in *Play Misty For Me*. In *Screening the Male: Exploring Masculinities in Hollywood Cinema*, ed. Steven Cohan and Ina Rae Hark. New York: Routledge, pp. 87-102.

KNIGHT, A. (1974). Playboy interview: Clint Eastwood. *Playboy*, 21: 57-58.

NEALE, S. (1993). Masculinity as spectacle: reflections on men and mainstream cinema. In *Screening the Male: Exploring Masculinities in Hollywood Cinema*, ed. Steven Cohan and Ina Rae Hark. York: Routledge, pp. 9-20.

SMITH, P. (1993). *Clint Eastwood: A Cultural Production*. Minneapolis, MN: Univ. of Minnesota Press.

16. THE THING FROM INNER SPACE: *TITANIC* AND *DEEP IMPACT*

SLAVOJ ZIZEK, LJUBLJANA

Let us recall the opening scene of *Star Wars*: at first, all we see is the void—the infinite dark sky, the ominously silent abyss of the universe, with dispersed twinkling stars that are not so much material objects as abstract points, markers of spatial co-ordinates, virtual objects; then, all of a sudden, in Dolby stereo, we hear a thundering sound coming from behind our backs, from our innermost background, later rejoined by the visual object, the source of this sound—the gigantic spaceship, a kind of space version of the *Titanic*—which triumphantly enters the frame of screen-reality. The object-Thing is thus clearly rendered as a part of ourselves that we eject into reality. This intrusion of the massive Thing seems to bring relief, cancelling the *horror vacui* of staring at the infinite void of the universe; however, what if its actual effect is the exact opposite? What if the true horror is that of Something—the intrusion of some excessive massive Real—where we expect Nothing? This experience of 'Something (the stain of the Real) instead of Nothing' may be at the root of the metaphysical question 'Why is there something instead of nothing?'

How does this traumatic Thing relate to the libidinal economy of the subjects affected by it? Let us begin with James Cameron's *Titanic*: not only is the *Titanic* a Thing *par excellence*, a mysterious object dwelling in the deep of the ocean, so that when human beings

approach it and take photographs of it, this disturbance of the peace
of the wreck is experienced as the transgressive entry into a forbidden domain; perhaps the key to the film's success is the way in which
it implicitly relates the Thing to the deadlocks of sexual relationship. In contrast to the standard catastrophe story, in which the
onset of something like an earthquake or floods allows people to
overcome their narrow conflicts and generates new global social
solidarity, the catastrophe in *Titanic* brings to light subterranean
social tensions between higher and lower classes—it is after the
catastrophe that these tensions fully explode. But, again, we see how
this is framed by the topic of the production of a couple. The
moment of the accident is crucial here: it occurs directly after the
sexual act, as if the crash is a punishment for the (sexually and
socially) transgressive act. More precisely, the crash occurs when
Rose proclaims that in New York she will abandon her old life and
join Jack—of course, this would have been the true catastrophe, the
ultimate disappointment (could she effectively live happily with
him, a vagabond without a proper home or financial means?). Thus,
it is as if the iceberg hits the ship and the catastrophe occurs in order
to prevent/occlude the much stronger libidinal catastrophe/disap-
pointment of two lovers happily being together and then seeing
their union degenerate. This is Hollywood at its purest: the catastrophe (iceberg hitting the ship) is reinterpreted as an answer of the
Real to the deadlock of the creation of the couple. The creation of
the heterosexual love-couple is the ultimate hermeneutic frame of
reference for the meaning of the film.

Against this background, one can also properly locate one of the
surprisingly refined moments in *Titanic*, which occurs when Jack

passes away in the freezing water, with Rose safe on a floating piece of wood, desperately clutching his hands. Realising that she is holding a corpse, Rose exclaims: 'Nothing can take us apart! I'll never let you go!' However, the act that accompanies these pathetic words is the opposite gesture of *letting him go*, of gently pushing him away, so that he gets sucked into the dark water.

Rather than a complete lover, Jack is then a kind of vanishing mediator for Kate: when her ego is shattered, he restores her mirror-image to her (by literally drawing her idealised image), and then, after sacrificing himself fully for her, and giving her final instructions ('You will have a lot of children, lead a long life ...'), graciously disappears into the abyss of the ocean and so erases himself from the picture. So, more than a story of the constitution of the couple, *Titanic* is a film about the restoration of the full narcissistic self-image of a woman. Rose identifies herself after her survival to the officer as 'Rose Dawson', accepting *his* name. However, the problem with this is not so much that her liberation is identified with the assumption of the male name, but that *he* had to die for this to be possible. So there is a limit to Cameron's Hollywood Marxism: the closing scene repeats the one in which Jack approaches Rose on the luxurious staircase to attend the first-class dinner to which he is invited for saving her, but this time it is a classless dream; passengers from all classes, from the Captain to the third-class immigrants, watch the couple unite and applaud them, with Jack dressed in his normal working-class attire. Although it is tempting to admire the simple beauty and cinematic efficiency of this final scene, we learn that after the catastrophe Rose continues to lead an upper-class life—Jack is just a 'vanishing mediator' to be rejected after he

has fulfilled his mission of liberating her from the suffocating con-
straints of her class prejudices. At the end, the old Rose throws the
big diamond into the sea: throughout the film, the problem is that of
accepting the loss of some precious object as the price of becoming
mature, and, ultimately, this object is Jack himself whose disappearance in the depths is correlative with the disappearance of the diamond. This, then, also accounts for the fact that, when the ship
sinks, the couple jump into the sea from the very place (the extreme
stern of the ship) from which Rose wanted to jump when Jack
approached her for the first time and pretended to be ready to join
her in her jump in order to dissuade her from doing it. Her first
jump would have been the suicidal attempt of an immature, spoiled
and disappointed brat, while her second jump, together with Jack,
involves a mature person's decision to embrace life.

This Freudian reading of a catastrophe as the reification of some
disturbance in sexual relationship seems to work also in the cases
where the Thing is an intruder from outer space. In the latest in the
series of cosmic catastrophe films, Miami Leder's *Deep Impact*
(1998), the Thing is a gigantic comet threatening to hit the Earth
and to extinguish all life for two years. At the end, the Earth is saved
by the heroic suicidal action of a group of astronauts with atomic
weapons; only a small fragment of the comet falls into the ocean east
of New York, causing a colossal wave, hundreds of yards high, that
flushes the entire north-east coast of the USA, inclusive of New
York and Washington. This comet-Thing also creates a couple, but
an unexpected one: the incestuous couple of the young, obviously
neurotic, sexually inactive TV reporter (Tea Leoni) and her promis-
cuous father (Maximilian Schell), who has divorced her mother and

just married a young woman of the same age as his daughter. It is clear that the film is effectively a drama about this unresolved proto-incestuous father–daughter relationship: the threatening comet obviously gives body to the self-destructive rage of the heroine, without a boyfriend, with an obvious traumatic fixation on her father, flabbergasted by her father's remarriage, unable to come to terms with the fact that he has abandoned her for her peer. The President (played by Morgan Freeman, in a politically correct vein), who, in a broadcast to the nation, announces the looming catastrophe, acts as the ideal counterpoint to the obscene real father, as a caring paternal figure (without a noticeable wife!) who, significantly, gives her a privileged role at the press conference, allowing her to ask the first questions. The link of the comet with the dark, obscene underside of paternal authority is made clear through the way the heroine gets in touch with the President. In her investigation, she discovers an impending financial scandal (large-scale illegal government spending) connected with 'ELLE'—her first idea, of course, is that the President himself is involved in a sex scandal, i.e. that 'Elle' refers to his mistress; she then discovers the truth. It turns out that 'E.L.E' is a codename for the emergency measures to be taken when an accident that could lead to total extinction of life threatens Earth, and the government has secretly been spending funds building a gigantic underground shelter in which one million Americans will be able to survive the catastrophe.

The approaching comet is thus clearly a metaphoric substitute for paternal infidelity, for the libidinal catastrophe of a daughter facing the fact that her obscene father has chosen another young woman over her. The entire machinery of the

global catastrophe is thus set in motion so that the father's
young wife will abandon him, and the father will return not to
his wife, the heroine's mother, but to her daughter. The culmina-
tion of the film is the scene in which the heroine rejoins her
father who, alone in his luxurious seaside house, awaits the
impending wave. She finds him walking along the shoreline;
they make peace with each other and embrace, silently awaiting
the wave; when the wave approaches and is already casting its
large shadow over them, she draws herself closer to her father,
gently crying 'Daddy!', as if to seek protection in him, reconsti-
tuting the childhood scene of a small girl safeguarded by the
father's loving embrace, and a second later they are both swept
away by the gigantic wave. The heroine's helplessness and vulnerability in this scene should not deceive us. She is the evil
spirit who, in the underlying libidinal machinery of the film's
narrative, pulls the strings, and this scene of finding death in the
protective father's embrace is the realisation of her ultimate
wish. The scene on the waterfront with the gigantic wave sweeping away the embraced daughter and father is thus to be read
against the background of the standard Hollywood motif (rendered famous in Fred Zinneman's *From Here to Eternity*) of the
couple making love on the beach, brushed by waves (Burt Lan-
caster and Deborah Kerr). Here, the couple is the truly deadly
incestuous one, not the straight one, so the wave is the gigantic
killing wave, not the modest shake of small beach waves.

Interestingly enough, the other big 1998 blockbuster-variation
on the theme of a gigantic comet threatening Earth, *Armageddon*,
also focuses on the incestuous father–daughter relation. Here, how-

ever, it is the father (Bruce Willis) who is excessively attached to his daughter: the comet's destructive force gives body to his fury at his daughter's love affairs with other men of her age. Significantly, the *dénouement* is also more 'positive', not self-destructive: the father sacrifices himself in order to save Earth, i.e. effectively—at the level of the underlying libidinal economy—erasing himself from the picture in order to bless the marriage of his daughter with her young lover.

From all these cases, we can see that beneath the multiple ways in which the Thing relates to the interpersonal libidinal relations there is a common matrix. That is, beneath the catastrophe of the Thing as a blessing in disguise, an intrusion that prevents another, true, catastrophe, the intrusion of the catastrophic Thing as the signal and/or payment for some social-sexual transgression—ultimately, the Thing as the direct embodiment of an incestuous transgression—there is the contradictory logic that characterises the working of the Unconscious, the intrusion of the Thing stands for the sexual (ultimately incestuous) transgression and, simultaneously, for the punishment for this transgression. This transgression, of course, relates to the failure of the 'normal' resolution of the oedipal constellation—from all these cases, it is thus clear that, far from belonging to a bygone era, the oedipal scenario is alive and well in today's popular culture.

17. *CHINATOWN*

NOEL HESS, London

As is often true for the patient's first words in a session, the opening image of Polanski's *Chinatown* (1974) sets the scene for the particular psychological terrain that the film will explore. The first thing we see is a photograph of a sexual couple. Clearly, the couple, caught in an act of private passion, have been seen by a hidden third party, the photographer. A series of photographs depicts the intercourse. This is accompanied by a moaning sound from the person (as yet unseen) who is looking at, or being shown, these photographs. There is a momentary ambiguity—is it a moan of voyeuristic excitement or of jealous agony? Quite quickly, the conventions and context of the scene are established. The photographs are being shown by a 'private eye' to the husband of the woman photographed. The husband is in a rage, and says, in almost the first words we hear: 'She's just no good', and soon after, 'I think I'll kill her'.

While the initial ambiguities resolve into a conventional situation, one we feel familiar with within the genre, it is important to hold on to that initial strangeness, because it does throw us into the situation of the primal scene, of oedipal rage at the sexual mother and the private eye that watches. *Chinatown* will explore this territory of incestuous longings, and subtly contrast it with actual incest. In an important contribution Simon (1992) has shown how, in what he describes as 'the history of an error', these two radically different but related situations are often muddled, both in our thinking and in the history of psychoanalysis. He compares incest survivors with Holocaust survivors, and by almost equating incest or sexual abuse (and it is interesting to note how the latter term has now replaced the former) with oedipal urges, psychoanalysis has done a serious disservice to the real and devastating trauma of incest. The main character of *Chinatown*, the private eye, J. J. Gittes, makes a similar mistake, with equally devastating effects, by becoming drawn into a sexual relationship, because of his own oedipal desires, with an abused and damaged object. His attraction to her is oedipal because she is the exclusive possession of the man who has abused her.

Gittes is profoundly shocked to discover that the woman he is protecting (Evelyn Mulray), whom he is in love with and wants to possess, had an incestuous relationship with her father (Noah Cross) during her adolescence, which produced a daughter. This admission is brutally beaten out of her, although there is some evidence that Gittes may, or could, already know this but is unable to face it, preferring to turn a blind eye to this sexual couple of father and daughter. Like Oedipus, he sees and does not see an incestuous crime (Steiner, 1985). He knows that her father (Noah Cross, whose name suggests duplicity, as well as the oedipal crossroads) is a powerful, ruthless and destructive man who believes that he possesses his daughter, and was in fact a business partner of her husband (reinforcing the sense of incestuous ties). She explicitly warns Gittes that her father is 'a very dangerous man', and adds, 'you may think you know what's going on, but you don't'. Her father had said exactly the same thing to Gittes at a previous meeting between them when they discussed his daughter, who Cross describes (with painful irony) as 'a very disturbed woman ... I don't want her taken advantage of'. When Evelyn finally confesses the fact of her incest to Gittes, and forces him to face it, she says, 'My father and I ... understand? ... or is it too tough for you?'

It is indeed too tough for him. Prior to this, Gittes fails to hear what is being hinted about the nature of this relationship between father and daughter because of his own inner blindness. Eyes are a crucial motif in the film, in two main forms. Firstly, there is the intrusive and voyeuristic private eye. We see how skilled Gittes is at gathering information by cunningly and intrusively gaining access to official departments, and rifling secretly through desks and drawers (Eaton, 1997). This is the eye that wants to see, but equally there is the recurring symbol in the film of the eye that cannot see. Gittes is attacked by farmers in an orange grove, and has one eye of his sunglasses knocked out. When he follows Evelyn's car, he smashes one of the car's tail-lights to make it easier to follow in the dark. Gittes finds out that Noah Cross has killed Evelyn's husband by finding Cross's broken glasses in a pool of water. Evelyn has a 'flawed eye', 'something black in the iris', as Gittes describes it (symbolising her incest), and she is shot through this flawed eye at the end of the film. It is in fact immediately after the discovery of her flawed eye that they kiss for the first time, as though her flawed eye has given Gittes a point of unconscious identification with her. For he, too, has a flawed eye, and cannot see what is in front of him until it is too late, because such knowledge is 'too tough'.

Gittes cannot see what he is caught up in, and thus cannot foresee where it will lead—to Chinatown, and the death of the woman

he loves. We know this because he has told us it has happened
before. As he tells Evelyn, when he was a cop on the beat in Chinatown, 'I thought I was trying to keep someone from being hurt, and
actually I ended up making sure they were hurt'. To clarify, Evelyn
asks: '*Cherchez la femme?* Was a woman involved? Is she dead?' The
phone rings, and the question is, ominously, left unanswered.
Although Gittes puts this disaster down to 'bad luck ... you can't
always tell what's going on', the way his account is phrased clearly
indicates some awareness of the unconscious motivation—that he
wanted the woman he loved to be killed. But why? Because, perhaps,
he knows that he can never possess Evelyn, that she is inextricably
tied to her father as a result of their sexual relationship, that her
father has destroyed her and she will never be free of him. Gittes
knows that if he brings a woman to Chinatown she will be killed,
and this is the compulsion he is condemned to repeat.

The Oedipus tale, we need to remember, is a story of an actual
incestuous relationship, which Freud universalised to describe
longings and conflicts that are a crucial aspect of normal development. The original myth, however, describes the devastating results
of actual incest—plague, murder, self-mutilation, suicide. The Los
Angeles of *Chinatown* is in the grip of a drought, which, like the
plague in Thebes, is an external manifestation of an inner disaster.
Noah Cross steals water from the city to irrigate land he plans to
own, just as he stole his daughter's sexuality. Water is essential for
life, and Cross can be seen to be stealing life, which he justifies with
a kind of psychotic omnipotence: 'Most people don't have to face the
fact that, at the right time and the right place, they are capable of
anything'. This is said to Gittes in a messianic, triumphant justifica-

tion of his incest but, if the same words are heard without the triumphant note, they suggest a different meaning—that such evil is in
fact universal. Gittes fails to hear this other meaning, which might
warn him of his own capacity for destructiveness. Gittes, like his
client to whom he shows the photographs at the beginning of the
film, is forced to look at the evidence of a sexual couple, from which
he is excluded, and this exclusion provokes murderous impulses.

Though not the only examples of violence in the film, there is
nevertheless a dominant theme of violence directed towards the
organs of perception. Evelyn is shot through her eye, Gittes has a
knife inserted in his nostril, and one of Cross's henchmen puts a
gun in Gittes's ear. As well as a violent representation of intercourse, these attacks seem to convey a wish to obliterate the most
basic means we have to acquire knowledge, through sensation and
perception, so as to keep us deaf, dumb, blind and ignorant of the
truth. Although these attacks come from various sources, including from an omnipotent destructive object (Noah Cross), they can
be seen as the depiction of a process that actively attacks the capacity to know, preferring psychic blindness. Gittes says to a woman
client who wants him to investigate her husband's adultery: 'Do
you know the expression "let sleeping dogs lie"? You're better off
not knowing'.

Chinatown, the place, has many meanings. It evokes something
sinister, exciting, dangerous, primitive and alien—the place where
things that should not happen do happen. It is a place of cruelty,
murderousness and sexual betrayal. The punch-line of a joke
Gittes tells his colleagues (and which he is tremendously excited
by) has a wife tell her husband, 'You're screwing like a Chinaman!'

This particular kind of intercourse, as the joke elaborates, is cruel, prolonged and interrupted. But the point of the punch-line is the revelation that the wife has actually been screwed by a Chinaman, and Gittes's excitement is because this betrayal is exposed: Chinatown is a place where the sexual mother and her betrayal is exposed. Chinatown is also a place where Gittes has previously brought about a tragedy, an experience from which he has learned nothing. It is the place in which, as he tells Evelyn, he was advised previously to do 'as little as possible', advice he again ignores and brings about a second tragedy. He almost incoherently mumbles these same words at the end of the film as he looks with horror at the murdered body of the woman he loved, finally comprehending, perhaps, what he has been condemned to repeat. 'She's no good ... I think I'll kill her.' These words echo in our mind from the beginning of the film, and we come full circle to that very wish enacted. Chinatown, finally, is the place of convergence of Gittes's oedipal wishes with the catastrophic fact of actual incest with its accompanying burden of intolerable guilt and psychic damage.

Auden (1963) has described the detective story as a dialectic between innocence and guilt. *Chinatown* plays interesting tricks with this dialectic by presenting the detective, who appears initially to be as sophisticated and cynical as he believes himself to be, as in fact unable to see the crucial truths that are in front of him. The writer of *Chinatown*, Robert Towne, makes this very point:

'In a classic detective story, generally speaking, the hero, like Oedipus, shares to some extent the responsibility for the crime, by either a failure to see it or hubris of some kind that he can solve a problem. In attempting to solve it, he becomes part of the problem ... In a classic detective movie ... where the detective is the kind of central figure involved in an investigation, he is really investigating his own limits to act in a way that is meaningful and positive' (Towne, 1996, pp. 114–5).

It is this failure that forcefully and painfully confronts Gittes at the climax of the film. Instead of doing 'as little as possible' (describing, perhaps, analytic neutrality), the only safe response to the dangerous world of Chinatown, Gittes has been seduced into action, into enacting a rescue fantasy that is perhaps unconsciously motivated by murderous impulses masked by the 'hubris' (i.e. omnipotence) Towne describes above.

It may be argued that a detective has no business being 'neutral' when his job is to save, rescue, apprehend etc. However, what makes *Chinatown* so interesting and moving compared with many other examples of the *film noir* genre (to which it mostly conforms, despite taking place in Californian sunshine) is that Gittes is unable to comprehend the dangerous limitations of action in a place where he knows from experience that doing 'as little as possible' is the only sane and safe response. According to this reading of the film, the final crime is his own.

By the end, the 'guilty' man (Cross) goes free, the 'victim' (Evelyn) is killed, and the 'innocent' man (Gittes) is horrified by having apparently inadvertently brought this about. Indeed, the climax of the film can be read as an account of the various ways in which unbearable guilt is dealt with. Each of the main characters embodies a different pathway. Cross psychotically and omnipotently denies guilt. He steals away the girl who is the product of his incest and evades justice. Evelyn, like Jocasta and Oedipus, achieves punishment for her crime through blindness and death. In a sense, her death is as much an unconscious suicide as a murder. Gittes, however, has to live with what has happened, and with what he has, in part, brought about. The expression on his face at the end of the film fully conveys the appalling horror of having to bear this emotional pain. The famous last line of the film—'Don't worry, Jake, it's just ... Chinatown'—is complex and ambiguous. Superficially, it suggests a certain invitation complacently to blame the external situation. However, at a deeper level, it conveys a need for the awareness of the inevitability of the compulsion to repeat destructive enactments.

REFERENCES

AUDEN, W. H. (1963). The guilty vicarage. In *The Dyer's Hand and Other Essays*. London: Faber, pp. 146–58.

EATON, M. (1997). *Chinatown*. London: BFI Film Classics.

SIMON, B. (1992). 'Incest—see under Oedipus complex'. The history of an error in psychoanalysis. *J. Amer. Psychoanal. Assn*, 40: 955–88.

STEINER, J. (1985). Turning a blind eye: the cover-up for Oedipus. *Int. J. Psychoanal.*, 12: 161–72.

TOWNE, R. (1996). On writing. In *Projections 6*, ed. J. Boorman and W. Donoghue. London: Faber, pp. 114–15.

18. SAVING PRIVATE RYAN'S SURPLUS REPRESSION

KRIN GABBARD, NEW YORK

How did a film as conventional and predictable as Steven Spielberg's *Saving Private Ryan* (1998) find so warm a reception among so many Americans? I would suggest that the oedipal issues that have long underpinned Spielberg's work have led him once again to touch his viewers at an especially vulnerable spot in their unconscious minds.

Although commentators have repeatedly praised the twenty minutes of bloody combat that opens the film, it is the first three minutes of the D-Day re-enactment that are the most crucial. When the front of the first landing craft drops open, virtually all of the infantrymen in the boat are immediately hit with machine-gun fire. We then see several men jumping into the sea as they try to escape from another landing craft; two are shot underwater and a third drowns under the weight of his backpack and gear. These are the film's lasting images of the absurdity of war, exploding conventional notions of heroism and the role of the individual soldier in battle. At this point *Saving Private Ryan* seems to suggest that war is senseless slaughter. But after these first few minutes, the American soldiers in *Saving Private Ryan* begin to fight back, and we get to know them. For the rest of the film the slaughter ceases to be senseless. As in the vast majority of American war movies, the possibilities for heroism and the contribution of the individual soldier are constantly available. Spielberg departs from the more recent

paradigm of war films in the nineteen seventies and eighties by suggesting, unironically and sentimentally, that war is about building
character and not about senseless slaughter. The film joins other
recent projects in promoting conservative retrenchment through
nostalgia for World War II.

In this context, the figure who has been continually brought forth
to authenticate Spielberg's vision of war in general and of World
War II in particular is Stephen E. Ambrose, the author of a collection
of books about World War II that now amounts to a mini-industry.
Spielberg and Robert Rodat, who is credited with the film's screenplay, found many of the details for their script in Ambrose's work,
especially his best-selling books *Band of Brothers* (1993), *D-Day June
6, 1944* (1995) and *Citizen Soldiers* (1997). After Spielberg invited
Ambrose to a preview screening of *Saving Private Ryan*, Ambrose's
reaction to the opening battle scene was widely reported: he said that
he was so affected by the film's realism that he crawled under his seat
and asked the projectionist to stop for a moment.

One might think that Stephen Ambrose himself landed at Omaha
Beach on 6 June, 1944. In fact, Ambrose was born in 1936 and
knows the war only at second hand, mostly from the several hundred veterans he has sought out in his research. Significantly, in his
own autobiographical statements, Ambrose never reports accounts
of war from his father, a Navy flight surgeon during World War II.
I would speculate that the senior Ambrose is one of those veterans
who preferred not to talk about what happened to him during the
war. When the younger Ambrose interviewed the men who did
want to talk about it, their accounts were several decades old and
surely revised and elaborated, as is always the case with oral culture.

Nevertheless, Ambrose has apparently reproduced their stories without question; if he has edited the stories for his books, he does not say so. Even though he does not hesitate to catalogue the horrors of war, Ambrose consistently presents the same romantic view of American men in battle that we know so well from the Hollywood cinema. Surely Ambrose's subjects, like Ambrose himself, have seen a lot of war movies.

Stephen Ambrose has much in common with Steven Spielberg, who has also seen a lot of war movies, and whose father was a radio operator with a B-24 squadron in Burma during the war. Like Ambrose seeking out hundreds of veterans, Spielberg has obsessively returned to World War II throughout his career, with two of the Indiana Jones films (1981, 1989), with his one great comic experiment *1941* (1979), with *Empire of the Sun* (1987), with *Schindler's List* (1993), and even with *Always* (1989), a remake of *A Guy Named Joe* (1943), one of the most consoling films of World War II. As Harvey Greenberg (1991) has suggested, these films may have been Spielberg's way of working through his relationship with his father, just as Ambrose was probably engaged in something similar in his obsessive pursuit of World War II veterans.

Not surprisingly, Spielberg has idealised many of the American soldiers in *Saving Private Ryan*, especially Captain John Miller, the Tom Hanks character. In the opening scene, for example, Spielberg does not show the Captain repeatedly ordering men into certain death as officers did during the several hours that Americans worked their way up the beach on D-Day. Most of what Spielberg does show in *Saving Private Ryan* should be familiar to anyone who has watched war movies such as *The Steel Helmet* (1951), *Catch-22*

(1970) and *Full Metal Jacket* (1987). In *The Big Red One* (1980) director Samuel Fuller anticipated Spielberg by eighteen years when he
showed the legendary red tide on the shore at Omaha Beach.

What is new in *Saving Private Ryan* is the post-Vietnam project of
consolation and what Jacques Derrida would call 'guilty nostalgia'
for the war years. Unlike most of the infantrymen in World War II,
the men in *Saving Private Ryan* admire and protect their Captain. He
fits into an organic chain of command that stretches seamlessly up to
General George Marshall (Harve Presnell), who brings the moral
authority of Abraham Lincoln into an idealised headquarters clearly
inspired by Norman Rockwell. After the soft-focus, magisterial sin-
cerity of General Marshall in ordering the mission to save Private
Ryan, any cynicism expressed by anyone in the squad (or in the audience) sounds hollow. In those days, the film tells us (and unlike today,
the film implies), the system worked and morality was unambiguous.

Similarly, the film reassures us that war is, in fact, a test of manhood and courage and that a warrior aristocracy will naturally
emerge, even if Captain Miller has to take a moment to sob in private.
His heroism and that of the men in his squad is a sharp contrast to
the cowardice of Corporal Upham, the intellectual played by Jeremy
Davies, who, at least according to Richard Goldstein (1999), symbol-
ises the large group of baby boomers who sat out their war with II-S
deferments and refused to be tested in the crucible of battle.

The film is most consistent with the old cinematic myths when
Captain Miller dies. Up until this point, the film has shown us a
number of 'realistic' death scenes, including the bloody death of
Medic Wade (Giovanni Ribisi), who asks for morphine and then for
his mother as he expires. But when Captain Miller dies, he not only

dies a conventional, mostly bloodless movie death; he doesn't cry out for his mother, his wife, or even himself. Instead, he devotes his last words to dispensing life-changing advice to a man he barely knows. Like Presnell's George Marshall, Captain Miller is an ideal-ised paternal imago, filling in for the missing father of Private Ryan and his four lost brothers. The ubiquitous oedipal thematics of the film seem to demand that Miller expire after his otherwise inexpli-cable moment of fatherly attention to James F. Ryan.

Because of what may be a partially unconscious oedipal agenda of his own, Steven Spielberg has spent a good deal of his career trying to make sense of World War II, even experimenting with the giddy satire of *1941*. But with *Saving Private Ryan* he has idealised the war and the men who fought it, at a time when many Americans are experiencing the death of a parent or grandparent who played some role in that war. Tom Brokaw's *The Greatest Generation* (1998), part of the same ideological project, is the nation's number-one best-sell-ing non-fiction hardback book at the time of this writing. During the impeachment follies of late 1998 and early 1999, both Lindsay Graham and Henry Hyde invoked the men who fought for Amer-ica—especially the men who landed at Normandy on June 6—as they argued for the impeachment and removal of that best-known of all baby-boomer draft-dodgers, Bill Clinton.

For Steven Spielberg, Stephen Ambrose, Tom Brokaw, Lindsay Graham and the rest, insisting that World War II was the Good War is at the very least a means of reconciling with dying fathers who may have made real face-to-face reconciliation difficult. It is also an excellent example of what Herbert Marcuse has called 'sur-plus repression'. Americans are currently being asked to repress more than just oedipal hostility against fathers who fought in World War II. They are also being asked to repress the conviction that their society has improved since the passing of the Old Order that the fathers represent. Appropriately, in the world of *Saving Private Ryan*, white males go about their work unencumbered by affirmative action guidelines and civil rights laws, and they express their erotic fantasies about young women without guilt or self-consciousness. The film argues that the Good War was a necessary, life-defining experience that baby boomers and Generation X-ers will never know. A baby boomer himself, Steven Spielberg has struck it rich once again, even as he paints his own generation as a group of hollow men standing in the shadows of their fathers.

REFERENCES

AMBROSE, S. E. (1993). *Band of Brothers: E Company, 506th Regiment, 101st Airborne from Normandy to Hitler's Eagle's Nest.* New York: Touchstone Books.

—— (1995). *D-Day June 6, 1944: The Climactic Battle of World War II.* New York: Simon & Schuster.

—— (1997). *Citizen Soldiers: The U.S. Army from the Normandy Beaches to the Bulge to the Surrender of Germany, June 7, 1944–May 7, 1945.* New York: Simon & Schuster.

BROKAW, T. (1998). *The Greatest Generation.* New York: Random House.

GOLDSTEIN, R. (1999). World War II chic. *The Village Voice*, Jan. 19: 42–7.

GREENBERG, H. R. (1991). Raiders of the lost text: remaking as contested homage in *Always. J. Popular Film & Television*, 18: 164–71.

19. $M(1931)^1$

JANINE CHASSEGUET-SMIRGEL, Paris

The premonitory character of Fritz Lang's *M* [*Mörder unter uns*] and its connection with the rise of Nazism has been indicated more than once. I would like to demonstrate the essential ambiguity in this linkage.

It is said that a masterpiece allows interpretations at multiple levels. According to Lang himself (though should we ever believe *auteurs?*), he just wanted to make a 'documentary' about a criminal and the process of police investigation. He tells us that he was inspired by *The Threepenny Opera* and by a news report about Berlin's organised crime mob searching for an unknown killer to get rid of the insistent presence of the police. To Lang then, the film is the hunt for a criminal and his subsequent judgement by the mob.

The Nazis themselves, already powerful enough in 1931 to dictate the law, forced Lang to change the original title of the film *Mörder unter uns* (Murderer[s] among us) to *M*, probably because they felt he was alluding to them! Rarely is a translated title better

---

[1] A paper concerning the same film was presented by the author at a colloquium organised in 1995 in Munich by Jochen Stork and published in 1998 (1: 61–9) in *Kinderanalyse*. The author is grateful to Jochen Stork for his permission to have this article reprinted in a modified version. This version was translated by Miguel A. Stamati.

than the original, but the alliteration in *M le Maudit* (M the cursed)[2] makes this more stirring than the original German title.

Although there had been the case of Peter Kürten, 'The Vampire of Düsseldorf', Lang and his wife, Thea von Harbou, co-authors of the screenplay, were inspired by the Grossman case in Berlin, as well as by other killers of children such as 'The Ogre of Hanover'.

The recurrence of this type of serial murder might be understood as a social symptom. Certainly, it is only in retrospect that these crimes, which appear to be isolated cases, make sense. In France the Weidman case is often brought to mind. Weidman killed at least seven people and was arrested on 9 December 1938. He was born in Frankfurt and executed in Versailles on 17 June 1939. This was the last public execution in France and it took place in the midst of unexpected agitation in the crowd, as if it were a premonitory event, heralding war, crime and the lawlessness of Nazism that would expand throughout Europe. This is a topic that Michel Tournier revisits in his 1970 novel *Le Roi des Aulnes* [The Erl-King].

Even a superficial reading of this film will focus on the individual psychology of the killer and the reactions of society, which is sufficient to keep one's interest. However, a second reading at least is called for. Even if we reject a purely socio-political reading of an oeuvre, the greatest creations cannot escape the context in which they were produced, just as dreams contain the day residues that contributed to their formation. We know that masterpieces are timeless, even if they draw their material from the context that gave them birth. We already find timelessness on a first reading of *M*: it is a fairy tale.

---

[2] *M* also stands for *meurtrier* [murderer].

M THE OGRE—A FAIRY TALE

From the beginning, *M* immerses us in the world of infantile imagination. The film starts with a human shadow crossed by an *M*, accompanied by the music of *Peer Gynt* (an interminable fairy tale). This theme, the only music played in the film, is whistled by M throughout the film. Then a counting-out rhyme starts, with the screen still black:

Warte, warte nur ein Weilchen
bald kommt der schwarze Mann zu dir,
mit dem kleinen Hackebeilchen
macht er Schabelfleisch aus dir.
Du bist raus !³

It is the story of the Ogre, of Saint Nicolas, of Hansel and Gretel, of the *Erl-King*. Behind the anxiety of the mothers (Elsie Beckmann's mother and the pregnant laundress) one can see the excitement of the girls playing. The Ogre and the *Erl-King* are irresistible seducers.

Spheres and circles punctuate the entire film and always appear linked to the child and her relation with M: the sphere of the pregnant woman's abdomen, the circle of children playing, Elsie's dance towards the signpost where the shadow of M is projected over the warning notice that promises a reward of one million marks for the capture of the murderer, the balloon that M buys for Elsie, Elsie's ball bouncing on uneven terrain (a sign that the crime has just been com-

---

³ Just you wait a little while/the nasty man will come/with his little axe/ he will chop you up/You are out!

mitted), M's fruit on his window-sill. Later we see the circles of the
police compass over the map of the city, M again slicing an apple in
front of the fruit stand with pineapples and grapefruits, M eating the
same apple in front of the showcase of the cutlery where his face is
reflected, together with the reflection of a new prey, the endless spiral
that the little girl looks into at the shop, next to the arrow that goes
up and down, the knife-penis of the impotent murderer. The little girl
is, this time, saved by the arrival of her mother. Then, again, another
little girl, the most seductive of them all, for whom M will buy sweets
in a store with the sign 'Obst und Südfrüchte' (regional and tropical
fruits). M peels an orange with his pocket-knife after buying the girl
a balloon like the one he bought for his first victim, sold by the same
blind beggar, while whistling the same melody of *Peer Gynt*, where he
fades out, singing 'in the castle of Halldu, king of the mountain ... '

When tales have a happy ending, the gnomes and the elves, the
spirits of the forest or a good fairy come to rescue the child. Here, it
is the Berlin mob that comes to the rescue. And the story doesn't
end there: it is like the endless spiral, or the eternal return of a circle
of children playing together. There will always be dark, dangerous
men attempting to seduce children and children who will let themselves be seduced. It was said that Peter Lorre (who plays M)
received hundreds of love letters after the film was shown.

In *Le Roi des Aulnes*, Michel Tournier writes that a warning is
directed to all mothers living in the regions of Gehlenburg, Sens-
burg, Lötzen and Lyck to beware the Ogre of Kaltenborn! The
hero, Tiffauges (the name of one of the castles of Gilles de Rais)[4]

---

[4] Friend of Jeanne d'Arc and murderer of children.

presents striking similarities with those he pretends to denounce. Ambiguity reigns.

M THE JEW

Another interpretation of the film is possible. When we see *M* today, our knowledge of history leads us to add meaning to the images. When we see the vertiginous staircase where Elsie's mother sees nothing to lessen her anxiety, we cannot help concluding that an intentional link is being made with the events still to come in Germany. The vast, bare attic and the clothes-lines on which some pieces of lingerie are hanging prefigure the dead bodies of children. And the power lines where the flying doll-shaped balloon gets caught make one think of the barbed wires of the concentration camps, even though we are in 1931. Although we should be prudent with our assumptions, we could say that the matrix of events to come is already present in the intuition of an artist. It is as fascinating for a historian as it is for a psychoanalyst to find in German books, works of art and films from the post-WWI era the intuitions of their creators foretelling the advent of Nazism.

Klein discovered fantasies of poisoning with gas (flatus), attacks with explosive excrement and burns from urine, as described in *The Psychoanalysis of Children* (1932), when she was in Berlin (1921 to 1926) for her analysis with Abraham.

In 1931, the breach between Jews and Germans is completed. M's trial by the mob takes place in the abandoned and tumbledown distillery *Kunz und Levi*, representing this breach, according to Ludwig Haessler (personal communication). It has often been said that the ranks of organised crime of Berlin, with its hierarchy, its laws, its courts (tribunals) already represented the Nazi party and its rise, a conclusion that is difficult to doubt. The boss, Schränker, played by Gustav Gründgens, with his leather trench-coat, his black gloves and his hat, reminds one irresistibly of the future members of the Gestapo, already present by then in the cadres of the Nazi party.

It is also difficult to separate what we know about Gründgens's[5] destiny (Klaus Mann made him the protagonist of his *Mephisto, History of a Career under the Third Reich* [1987]) from the character of Schränker and his words when he says about M: 'He must be eliminated, he must disappear, without pity' with accents that are properly Hitlerian. Perhaps, even there, one must recognise Lang's sensitivity in choosing Gründgens for this role.

But isn't M himself the epitome of the murderer, since he is a murderer of children? Was the title 'A murderer among us' (*Mörder unter uns*) an allusion to the Nazis? And would M then be the Nazi? The response cannot but be ambiguous. The real identity of Peter Lorre may influence us (his real name was Löwenstein). We have other clues: when M denounces himself in front of the mob tribunal as a cursed one, the carrier of a fire that burns, of a torment, is he not the Jew who supposedly killed Jesus Christ and who then was accused, throughout time and even today, in Russia and other parts, of killing Christian infants, of ritual killing, of putting the blood of infants in the unleavened bread for Passover?

---

[5] Gründgens, a Nazi party member, became an actor-fetish of the Third Reich cinema.

According to Gunnar Heinsohn in his book *What is Antisemitism?* (1978), the origin of anti-Semitism (or at least one of its roots) is in the prohibition in Judaism of the human sacrifice and of infant sacrifice in particular. ('You shall not sacrifice any infant of Moloch.' Thus God ended human sacrifices then commonly practised, replacing Isaac with a ram). He remarks that human sacrifice, especially infant sacrifice to the extent that Christ is equated with the infant-God, continues to be practised in the Christian religion, Catholic in particular, where the body and the blood of the Saviour are incorporated when there is belief in the 'real presence' during the Communion. In fact, there is a prohibition against incorporating blood in the Jewish ritual—the kosher diet prescribes that blood must be drained from meat and an egg that has been fertilised can't be eaten. One should underline the cannibalistic interdiction that these practices reflect. The Jew would then be an 'anti-Ogre', or, furthermore, the first one, no doubt, to oppose these practices and *ogresque* representations in others and in himself. In fact, one can understand the projection of infanticide on to the Jew as connected with the need to accuse the very one whose commandments prohibit it of a crime for which one is responsible.

If such is the case, M *would be the Jew on whom the secular accusation of infanticide is made.* And the film does nothing to withdraw this accusation. The theme of the circle, the sphere, the spiral, the ball, the balloon, which emerges throughout the film, is primarily a symbol of the foetus in the womb, as is the pregnant woman at the beginning of the film. *Avoir le ballon* is a colloquial French expression meaning 'to be pregnant'. At the same time, this sphere in the form of fruit that he eats is an illustration of M's ogre-like qualities.

Once the projection of the infanticide is made, the supposed murderer is marked by an *M* on the back, as the Jews will be marked by a yellow star, signalling the victim to be. However, even with the appeals of Schränker and the crowd ('We have to exterminate him, kill him like a dog'), there won't be an execution. The force will remain with the Law. The police will deliver M to Justice and a maternal voice off-camera will say towards the end: 'That won't give us our children back ... You'd better watch your children ...'

How do we understand this ending? Ambiguity here multiplies. 'In the name of the Law', says the voice of the policeman whose hand appears on M's shoulder. But, if this Law does not suffice to deliver us from the danger, is it then a matter of making use of another Law? If so, what Law then? Schränker's Law, perhaps, and the Law of the mob in general? Isn't this a call for emergency regulations that could get rid of M in a more efficient way than the one adopted by the impotent regime of the democratic Weimar Republic?

I can't help thinking that the *mise-en-scène* and the dialogues of this brilliant film have two authors, Fritz Lang and his wife at that time, Thea von Harbou. The former resisted Goebbels's offer to become the director of cinematography for the Third Reich and emigrated, on the very day of the invitation, to France and then to the US. Lang's wife, from whom he separated, later became a member of the Nazi Party. Perhaps the ambiguity of the film, especially of its ending, is a reflection in itself of these two divergent fates. Perhaps it is a reflection on the decaying Germany of the Weimar Republic. Perhaps the reflection of ourselves when we lack the courage to resist the ultimate vertigo of the irrational, when we have no father to protect us from the attraction of the *Erl-King* as we let ourselves fall under his fascinating and fatal dominion?

REFERENCES

HEINSOHN, G. (1978). *Was ist Antisemitismus?* Frankfurt: Eichborn.

KLEIN, M. (1932) *The Psychoanalysis of Children.* London: Hogarth.

MANN, K. (1987). *Mephisto, Histoire d'une carrière sous le IIIème Reich.* Paris: Denoël.

TOURNIER, M. (1970). *Le Roi des Aulnes.* Paris: Gallimard.

20. REMEMBERING AND REPEATING IN *EVE'S BAYOU*[1]

KIMBERLYN LEARY, ANN ARBOR, MI

In a Guest Editorial in the *International Journal of Psychoanalysis,* Glen Gabbard suggested that film 'speaks the language of the unconscious' (1997, p. 429). Films do their psychological work at the intersection of what is private and what is public. A film is effective when it taps into the hopes and fears of the audience and bridges the gap between private internal experience and collective psychology. In this way, the cinema serves as guardian both of personal subjectivity and public memory.

Kasi Lemmons's film *Eve's Bayou* occupies this divide between private reminiscence and public recollection. The film begins with an arresting voice-over: 'The summer I killed my father, I was 10 years old'. Told from the viewpoint of young Eve Batiste, the film is a haunting account of a black Creole family in the Louisiana bayou of 1962. It is a sequestered and self-contained world that few outsiders ever encounter. The Batiste family—descended from a slave, also named Eve, who saved her master's life and then bore him sixteen mulatto children—live a life of relative privilege in this black-only realm of river and swamp.

---

[1] An earlier version of this work was presented at a meeting of the Association for Advancement of Psychoanalytic Thought at the Michigan Psychoanalytic Association.

Eve's father, Louis, is the town's physician. He is a handsome but reckless man who spurns his beautiful wife only to parade his affairs with married women under her nose.

At a summer party, Eve is witness to her mother's humiliation as Louis twirls his latest conquest, Matty Mereaux, across the dance floor. Eve herself burns with jealousy when her father turns his attention to her older sister, Cecily, whom he chooses for his next dance. Eve's mother can offer little comfort and instead seeks her own consolation in her adoring relationship with Eve's younger brother, Poe. Eve retreats to the barn where she falls into a fitful sleep, only to be awakened by the sight of her father making love with Matty Mereaux. Father and daughter strike a transgressive deal with each other as Eve barters her knowledge of her father's dalliance for his promise of a future dance of her own. But when Eve tells her sister Cecily what she saw, Cecily tells her she is mistaken and offers her a substitute story, repainting Eve's memory to save for herself, as well as for Eve, an image of their father as hero. Eve finds some solace with her Aunt Mozelle—a spiritual counsellor with the gift of 'sight': the ability to foretell everyone's future but her own ('that's the way it always is, blind to my own life').

Cecily, however, frantically tries to reclaim their father as her own. Her desperation finally rouses her mother, who intervenes to tell Cecily that only she will wait up at night for Louis's return. Cecily retreats into a world of her own making until she discloses to Eve that she and Louis have shared a lovers' kiss. Eve's desire for revenge leads her to a conjuring woman, Elzora, from whom she wishes to purchase a spell to use against her father. *En route*, Eve encounters Matty Mereaux's husband, Lenny, and in a stunning moment, casually betrays her father's infidelity. Certain that she knows her own mind, Eve refuses Elzora's suggestion of a nominal curse and demands his death. To Eve's horror, Elzora obliges her. Frightened at what she has wrought, Eve flees to her father, hoping to protect him, but Matty Mereaux's husband, Lenny, reaches him first. Lenny warns Louis to stay away from his wife but a drunk and defiant Louis claims a final word that he pays for with his life. Only later does Eve learn that what remains of Cecily's memory of her father's kiss is a kaleidoscope of sensations and images, defying integration. Eve discovers she shares with her Aunt the gift of 'sight'. She can foretell the future, but she cannot repossess the past. She must live with what she doesn't know. The Voodoo Queen, Marie LeVeaux, is buried in St Louis Cemetery Number 1, not far from the French Quarter of New Orleans. Her grave is adorned with chicken bones, feathers and offerings of food left by the faithful. In Creole culture, if the saints can't help you, then perhaps the sorcerer might. Seen through one lens, this represents a practical and adaptive turn of affairs. It is one of the multitude of strategies oppressed people have developed to defy the odds and keep hope alive in their communities.

Eve's Bayou tells something of a universal story, to be sure. It is an allegory of the secret lives we harbour within. Each of the players struggles with his or her subterranean self. Each is consumed by the urgencies of their passions and the insistent need for recognition. *Eve's Bayou* shimmers with desire—from the soul-murdering confusion of desire fulfilled when Cecily and Louis kiss, to the narcissistic pain of desire that is deferred, dismissed or otherwise rejected. In the film's relentless attention to the force of desire and the compromises we effect to manage it, the Batistes cohere as recognisably psychoanalytic selves.

Lemmons uses her film to illuminate the materiality of our internal wishful lives, showing us the myriad ways in which desire is made flesh. Wishes lead us here, rather than there, and render us always a little out of control. We see this most plainly when Eve seeks out the conjuring woman, Elzora. Even before she finds Elzora, Eve betrays her father to Lenny Mereaux. Without fully realising it, Eve has cast her own spell and like Elzora's magic, it cannot be taken back.

At its centre, *Eve's Bayou* remains a very sophisticated meditation on the nature of memory—and its disturbances. 'I'm going to tell you what happened', says Cecily, walking Eve back to the moment of her encounter with Louis and Matty Mereaux. Lemmons dramatises for us the constructive nature of memories, the way we assemble them from our wishes, needs and attempts at self-justification. This is the territory of contentious debate. The controversies over repressed memory and childhood sexual abuse remain contested sites of theory and clinical practice. 'Now you believe me?' asks Eve, later in the film, her memory of Louis and Matty obviously intact. With this, Lemmons takes on the crucial issue of whether we are prepared to believe our children when they, like Eve, tell us things that we do not wish to hear.

Thus far, *Eve's Bayou* tells a familiar psychoanalytic story. It is, however, a film with a unique African-American sensibility. What makes the film *black*?

Hollywood films typically commercialise black bodies rather than explore black minds. In this respect, *Eve's Bayou* offers a picture of African-American subjectivity that is otherwise invisible. Or does it? The film critic, Alex Patterson, commented in an on-line review in 1998 that it was odd seeing a film about African-Americans in which there were no white folks, and not a single mention of race.

I think that Patterson got it wrong. I see Lemmons's film as offering an important and powerful commentary on the racial politics of contemporary America. If psychoanalysis teaches nothing else, it continually impresses upon us the way in which that which is absent is never gone but has only moved underground.

American racism is the absent presence of *Eve's Bayou*. At the start of the film, 'Gran Mere', Louis's mother, receives the compliment—'You must be so proud. Your son is the best coloured doctor in Louisiana'. Not the *best* doctor, but the best *coloured* doctor. It is a simple statement but one that speaks volumes about the impingement of the white world on the black psyche, even in the bayou.

Louis seems to understand this and to have bent himself to this social reality as we learn in the film's *dénouement* 'I'm only a small town doctor, pushing aspirin to the elderly. But to a certain type of woman, I'm a hero. I *need* to be a hero some time'. Louis effects for himself a narcissistic solution to the narcissistic problem forced upon him by a dominant culture so malignantly devaluing of black achievement. Louis's problem is clearly his own, even as it derives in part from something beyond his individual psychodynamics. The pressures imposed by a culture on to individuals are always complex and contradictory and always have unpredictable rather than uniform effects (Layton, 1998).

Louis tries to save himself in the arms of his many lovers, where he is able to reassure himself that he is a hero even though this self-same act of attempted self-preservation destroys his family. Turning passive into active, Louis taunts Lenny Mereaux to his breaking point, and thereby has a hand in his own demise. As the shot is fired, Louis pushes Eve out of harm's way, never knowing the guilt she is destined to bear forever as a result of her effort to repair her narcissistic wounds with her visit to Elzora.

It is possible that Lemmons offers the viewer a specifically racial perspective through the character of Elzora who has a white face when we are first introduced to her. What is the function of this detail? It is in the white face that Elzora calls Eve a thief, denounces her Aunt Mozelle as cursed and implies that Louis is no damn good. Could Elzora be the symbol of a white world that constructs black subjects as depraved, deficient and defective?

The truth is that we don't really know. Elzora does most of her dirty work without her mask, snatching money from Eve and violating her by forcing her to treat her wishes as fixed and certain realities ('you said you was sure'). What we do know is that of the four hundred films released by American studios in 1997, Kasi Lemmons was the only African-American woman director among them. 'The people making decisions make movies about what they want to see,' says Helena Echegoyen, a former executive at Miramax Films (Samuels & Leland, 1998). And what the film companies want to see rarely includes the complex subjectivity that Lemmons brings to life in *Eve's Bayou*.

In the end, the film forces us to confront the limits of our abilities to understand ourselves with the clarity we sometimes associate with going to the movies. We don't know what happened between Louis and Cecily, though we know undeniably that something did. We are left with a much-needed respect for the complexity of black minds and hearts. Perhaps this is more than enough for any one film.

Acknowledgement: This essay is dedicated to the memory of Mrs Ethel Goodreaux.

REFERENCES

GABBARD, G. (1997). The psychoanalyst at the movies (Guest Editorial). *Int. J. Psychoanal.*, 78: 429–34.

LAYTON, L. (1998). *Whose that boy? Whose that girl? Clinical Practice meets Postmodern Gender Theory*. Northvale, NJ: Aronson.

SAMUELS, A. & LELAND, J. (1998). Waiting to prevail. *Newsweek*, 12 January, 1998.

21. WATCHING VOYEURS: MICHAEL POWELL'S *PEEPING TOM* (1960)[1]

ANDREA SABBADINI, London

Looking, and being looked at, play important roles in the establishment and maintenance of interpersonal relationships. Of course, to state that all of us are therefore voyeurs would be an unnecessary generalisation because 'scopophilia' (or 'voyeurism') as a nosological category involves a libidinal over-investment in watching others that often replaces, rather than complements, other forms of emotional, physical or sexual contact. Yet, on account of our polymorphously perverse infancy, such a statement could equally be considered a commonplace. We psychoanalysts, furthermore, make ourselves particularly vulnerable to being labelled as voyeurs (though of the auditory rather than the visual kind), in so far as our profession also implies a curiosity about, or even a probing into, our analysands' internal worlds, including their darkest fantasies and secret passions.

Remembering Freud's observation that in its preliminary stage the scopophilic drive is autoerotic ('it has indeed an object, but that object is part of the subject's own body' [1915, p. 130]—this situation being the source of both voyeurism and exhibitionism), I would like to add that we can identify two contrasting and complementary

[1] This essay was presented on 14 December 1999 at the 'Freud at the threshold of the 21st century' Conference in Jerusalem (Israel).

kinds of voyeurism. The first one, which I shall call 'covert voyeurism', involves gratification, in the absence of exhibitionistic objects,
through the secretive, furtive, intrusive watching of others who are
unaware of being looked at: such as the girl followed by a man hiding
in the dark; but also the targets of professional spies and aptly
named private eyes (themselves the subjects, interestingly enough,
of two of the most popular film genres). The second form of scopophilia, which I shall call 'collusive voyeurism', involves on the
other hand gratification through gazing at people who are themselves aware of being watched—such as strippers in nightclubs; or,
indeed, any performers on stage—and who may themselves get
exhibitionistic satisfaction from being looked at.

These two kinds of scopophilia may not be incompatible, in the
sense that the same subject may get visual pleasure from either situation, but they are intrinsically different in their phenomenological
and psychogenetic features: covert voyeurism is a predatory form of
aggressivity, it is narcissistic, pregenital, more directly related to
primitive primal-scene phantasies and often experienced as shame-
ful. Collusive voyeurism, on the other hand, is a form of perversion
and it implies a more advanced level of development, and some recognition that others are not just extensions of one's selves, but
objects in their own right (even if they are often experienced and
treated simply as part-objects); and this is because their awareness
of the subject's voyeuristic activity is a requirement for his, or less
often her, gratification. It might also be of theoretical and clinical
interest to differentiate normal from pathological scopophilia. For
instance, it could be argued that a certain amount of collusive
voyeurism, probably modelled on the earliest exchanges of glances

between mother and baby at the breast, is present in all normal sexuality.

If we now narrow down our field of vision, we could magnify it on the specific sense in which we might describe ourselves as voyeurs at the cinema—or, more appropriately, *film-lovers*. According to Christian Metz, what is peculiar to cinema is not only that it allows us to perceive our object from a distance (through the senses of sight and hearing), but also that 'what remains in that distance is now no longer the object itself, it is a delegate' (1974, p. 61). We have here a perverse situation whereby while 'the actor was present when the spectator was not [during the shooting of the film], the spectator is present when the actor is no longer [during its projection]: a failure to meet of the voyeur and the exhibitionist' (p. 63). I should add here that my distinction between covert and collusive voyeurism corresponds to two different perspectives, also noticed by Metz, on the relationship between films and their spectators. From the former viewpoint, films are not exhibitionistic objects: they do not watch us, so to speak, watching them. From the latter, films are exhibitionistic objects, since being watched is the very purpose of their existence.

When the film in question—like Michael Powell's *Peeping Tom* (1960)—is about voyeurism itself, we find ourselves faced with an intriguing situation: because we are no longer just indulging in the scopophilic activity of watching a film, with all the wishes, anticipation, pleasure or disappointments intrinsic to such an activity. What we are watching now is other voyeurs like ourselves. In other words, our identifications and our visual excitement have as their objects not just the film itself, but also the subjects and objects of the

voyeuristic activities projected on the screen—a silver surface that
thus turns into the distorting mirror of our own suppressed desires.

When watching a film, is our point of view always located behind
the film-maker's camera? Does it necessarily coincide with that of
the protagonist? How much of ourselves is left sitting in the cinema's chair and how much of it is transported, as it were, on to the
screen? If there is an oscillation in this double register of identifications, when and why does it take place?

In the terrific opening sequence of *Peeping Tom*,[2] Michael Powell
places us in a fascinatingly paradoxical situation: not only behind
his own camera filming *Peeping Tom*, but also, collusively, behind
the viewfinder of the protagonist's half-hidden Super-Eight,
recording his own sadistic murders. Mark's camera is a phallic and
deadly weapon, literally 'shooting' its targeted preys, with the help
of its infernal paraphernalia: the sharpened tripod leg perforating
his victims' throats and the mirror reflecting their terrorised gazes
back to them. In the process, his essentially covert voyeurism is
turned into a collusive one—though here, of course, the objects are

---

[2] The protagonist, Mark, is a well-mannered psychopath, whom we
watch stabbing women to death with the tripod of his camera in order to
film their expression of terror. We learn that as a child he had been subjected to cruel experiments by his father, a biologist researching human
responses to fear. A young neighbour, Helen (Anna Massey), and her
wise blind mother, try unsuccessfully to understand his bizarre behaviour
and rescue him. In the final scene Mark, by now pursued by the police,
spectacularly kills himself in the same fashion in which he had murdered
his victims.

forced by his perversion into becoming exhibitionists against their wishes. Mark's victims—a prostitute, a model and an actress, whose activities already include a measure of narcissistic exhibitionism— are as vulnerable as he was himself as a child. The camera, and we suspect the projector as well, come then to represent the power of evil to seduce and destroy; the cinema screen becomes a looking- glass where we, the viewers, are made to witness our own wishes and fears reflected back at us in the characters with whom we iden- tify.

As we are propelled by the film into a no-man's-land between the two cameras, a splitting process is imposed on us whereby our visual and psychological place gets dislodged from what would otherwise be a more comfortable position. Such forced *dislocation* of perspective, and therefore of identification, and therefore of moral involvement, is what makes Powell's *Peeping Tom* so dis- turbing to us. This disturbance, I would suggest, is quite different from that induced by the *fragmentation* which characterises another classic film on voyeurism, Alfred Hitchcock's *Rear Win- dow* (1954). There the protagonist's fractured leg in a plaster cast (ambiguously both erect and impotent) becomes the starting- point for a series of further fragmentations that, ironically, provide the backbone to the whole film. In Jimmy Stewart's company we are coaxed into focusing our eyes, or binoculars or telephoto lens, on the multiple silent films framed by windows, simultaneously projected on to the apartments of his disturbingly over-normal neighbours. The fragmentations, both in content and form—of the main characters' identities, of the institution of marriage as society's supporting structure, of the architecture of the buildings and indeed of the film itself, plus the probable cutting into pieces of a female body—all contribute to our uncanny experience in front of the screen.

If we now return to Powell's film, we find that the grey area of dislocation that I have referred to is even more complex than it at first appears. For if it concerns an ambiguous oscillation between the spaces behind the two cameras, it also relates to a similarly ambiguous oscillation between the spaces in front of the two projectors: the one before our eyes when we watch *Peeping Tom*, and the one in Mark's darkroom. A dark room indeed! Half-hidden behind a thick curtain, this is no Winnicottian 'transitional space' of play and creativity, but a place, symbolic as it is real, representing (in spite of being located upstairs and not, contrary to our topographical expectations, in an underground cellar) the unconscious itself, full as it is of irrationality, repressed sexuality, deception and violence, and charged with intense primal-scene and pre-oedipal connotations. I will add that it is no coincidence that this room originally belonged to Mark's abusive father while, in contrast with it, the bedroom downstairs, which used to be his mother's, represents a less primitive and more oedipal space. It is here that Mark reluctantly lets Helen store his camera before they go out together for dinner. He knows that she, by removing his weapon, is castrating him of his murderous pregenital sexuality and replacing it with a potential for Romantic love—a condition desirable to her but terrifying to him because it challenges at its roots his own misogynous, predatory identity. We have learnt by now that Mark is irredeemable by Helen's innocent affection or, later, by the therapeutic efforts of her farsighted blind mother.[3] By daring to explore his lair—that is, by attempting to get closer to the darker corners of his mind—these Beauties only make themselves more vulnerable to becoming the Beast's next targets.

Peeping Tom presents us with an array of different forms of deviant sexuality and psychopathology: scopophilia, obsession with pornography, sadism and psychopathy, not to mention a deep depression underlying everything else. The cinematic gesture of linking them together in Mark's disordered personality seems to confirm Robert Stoller's view of perversion (indeed, of all sexuality) as being intrinsically characterised by a wish to humiliate and hurt: 'I found that hostility—the urge to harm one's sexual object—was a central dynamic' (1979, p. xii), he writes. Through the sexual act, 'frustration and trauma are converted to triumph, and, in fantasy, the victim of childhood is revenged' (p. 9).

Mark's voyeurism sadistically destroys his victims by literally penetrating them. It is clearly motivated by hatred, in contrast with the one we come across in another great film on this subject, Krysztof Kieslowski's *A Short Film About Love* (1988). There the protagonist's eyes, with prosthetic help from increasingly powerful optical instruments, let him travel the distance that separates his flat from that of a beautiful neighbour, and covertly penetrate her space with clumsy intrusiveness. Yet, as his initial masturbatory interest for her as a furtive object of instinctual gratification

---

[3] The blind seer is a *topos* derived from classical tragedy (e.g. Tiresias in Sophocles' *Oedipus Tyrannus* and present in other films too, e.g. Nicolas Roeg's *Don't Look Now*).

is replaced by love, even if doomed to tragedy, she stops being just a body to be watched and is gradually transformed, by his confession to her of his scopophilic activities, into a more real person now exhibitionistically colluding with his interest in her.

Mark's women instead, for all his charming manners, remain bodies to be hated. It is then understandable, much as it is regrettable, that *Peeping Tom* so unanimously enraged film critics when it opened in London in 1960: not so much because its content, gory without spilling a single drop of blood, was too morbid for its time; nor because of the pessimistic considerations one could draw from it about the function of cinema as a whole, also in view of the evidence, inconclusive as it may be, of the role sometimes played by distressing images in the perpetration of vicious crimes; but because being a film, in Martin Scorsese's words, 'where the process of film-making becomes an accessory to the crime' (1980), it stabbed the narcissistic film establishment at its heart by depicting both film-lovers and film-makers as voyeurs.

Using in places a melodramatic *mise-en-scène* that followed acceptable aesthetic conventions or lighting up the screenplay's dim subject with a healthy sense of self-referential flashes of humour, was not enough to save Powell's brilliant and prolific career (he was only to make three more films before his death in 1990). Nor was it helpful to him that he tried to give a psychological explanation to Mark's crimes by presenting them as cries of rage against his sadistic father, as well as rehearsals for his own approaching self-destruction. The excitement of fear is the driving force at the source of both Mark's and his father's perversions; and to produce documentaries on the effects of fright on its victims is the project that links them together, or rather ties them in an inextricable knot.[*] Powell's film thus indirectly raises questions about the long-lasting consequences of early parental influence. But does such a psychogenetic explanation, which equates Mark with the monstrous creation of a Frankenstein, also provide an ethical justification to his deeds? Is he—and indirectly we, as voyeuristic spectators—responsible? If in the end Mark's suicide on his own sword, or camera, in a pyrotechnic frenzy of flashbulbs, mirrors and audiotaped screams from his childhood, brings us spectators so much relief, it is because it allows us to avoid answering unbearable questions.

Films about voyeurism, such as *Peeping Tom*, give the medium of cinema an opportunity for self-reflection, which includes acknowledgement of responsibilities towards its spectators, as well as performing the cultural function of representing conflictual aspects of our inner reality and object relationships. A central role for cinema is to be a social provider of visual and auditory messages, which, not unlike psychoanalysis itself, can confirm our *Weltanschauung*, or challenge it at its very roots. Specifically in the emotionally loaded areas of sexual experience, identity and behaviour, and of the constantly shifting boundaries between normality and pathology, both psychoanalysis and cinema are enormously powerful languages that allow us—or, sometimes, even force us—to reconsider our assumptions, values and beliefs about ourselves.

---

[*] In the documentary Mark shows to Helen, it is Michael Powell and his son Columba who ironically, or some would say perversely, play the parts of the biologist and of Mark as a child.

REFERENCES

FREUD, S. (1915). Instincts and their vicissitudes. *S.E.* 14

METZ, C. (1974). The Imaginary Signifier. In *The Imaginary Signifier. Psychoanalysis and the Cinema.* Bloomington, IN: Indiana Univ. Press, 1982, pp. 1–87.

SCORSESE, M. (1980). Introduction to Michael Powell's *Peeping Tom.* London: British Broadcasting Corporation.

STOLLER, R. (1979). *Sexual Excitement. Dynamics of Erotic Life.* London: Maresfield Library.

22. EGOYAN'S *EXOTICA*:
WHERE DOES THE REAL HORROR RESIDE?[1]

RONIT MATALON AND EMANUEL BERMAN, Israel

'To me, the highest aim of any film is to enter so completely into the subconscious of the viewer that there are moments and scenes and gestures which can be generated by the spectator's imagination. That becomes part of the film they're playing in their mind, and I hope the film has enough space to allow that type of room, that type of exchange' (Egoyan, 1995, p. 50).

'What have we really seen?'

This question unites *Exotica*'s protagonists and *Exotica*'s viewers, who are at first mystified by the discontinuity and gaps between scenes. Visibility, and the impact of the visual image, are central themes of this film. Voyeurism, Egoyan implies, is not only a humiliating position of someone who cannot achieve more, cannot have 'the real thing': it also forms a relationship, and allows a unique position of power. By watching attentively one can influence the story, transform its sequence.

Is that why Francis's wife attempts to cover his camcorder lens with her hand, when he videotapes her and their daughter?

---

[1] An earlier version was presented at the Susan Zuckerman Memorial Program on 'Psychoanalysis and cinema', San Francisco, 22 April 2000. Ronit Matalon is a novelist; Emanuel Berman is a psychoanalyst.

The film opens at the airport, where customs inspectors watch the passengers through a one-way mirror; their gaze could determine a passenger's fate. We soon move to the 'Exotica' nightclub, where men watch the strippers, at times through a one-way mirror too. Francis (Bruce Greenwood) repeatedly watches a young stripper, Christina (Mia Kirshner), but their interaction appears highly ceremonial, built on set rules and steady mantras, which form a story co-constructed by the two of them. 'What would happen if someone ever hurt you?', he repeats; 'You'll always be there to protect me', she replies.

An additional central image is supplied by the pet shop owned by Thomas (Don McKellar), specialising in exotic animals. Seemingly, here we find the film's central motif: human beings as strange exotic animals, torn out of their natural habitat, forced to survive in an artificial aquarium-like reality, imitating their original milieu. 'Just because they are exotic doesn't mean they can't endure extremes. It is, after all, a jungle out there, isn't it?' says Francis, who comes as a tax inspector to check Thomas's books (once more, a penetrating fateful gaze). The Rousseau-styled artificial tropical vegetation of the 'Exotica' club portrays another such aquarium.

Yet, there is something deceptive in this too visible motive of exotic scopophilia directed at exotic fish-bowl visibility. If this were indeed the film's world view, we would be watching a slick commercial product, taking advantage of the linguistic cliché of the exotic, of the journalistic fascination with marginality and perversion. But the genuine emotional power of this film signifies Egoyan's capacity to critically deconstruct that popular image, and to allow the discovery of a moving human dimension behind it.

What Egoyan is fascinated by is not what people show and watch, but what people hide, or attempt to hide. 'You have to convince yourself that this person has something hidden that you have to find. You check his bags, but it's his face, his gestures, that you are really watching ...' explains the customs officer.

This dialogue between the images of visibility and what they disguise, between façade and tormented secrecy, between nudity and 'the privacy of the self', conveys also a dialectic Egoyan holds between postmodernist and modernist beliefs. He abundantly utilises the postmodernist fascination with visibility, façades, masks; with the arbitrary construction of roles. Imposture is a major theme in Egoyan's films: 'identity itself is malleable, to be borrowed, customized or invented' (Pevere, 1995, p. 18). And yet his protagonists painfully strive towards authentic meaning, and eventually appear to possess more of an inner core and of powerful, genuine emotions than we could initially know. ('What I find really fascinating is why emotions are repressed, why they are restrained, why they are held back. And people who were hurt by giving away too much emotion'; Egoyan, in *Current Biography*, 1994, p. 158). In this respect, this quintessential postmodernist film turns out to offer an antidote to any postmodernistic nihilism.

Exotica can also be seen as a critique of post-capitalist society. Buying emotional needs through money and possessions is a repetitive theme. The film outlines a complex network of exploitation, betrayal and blackmail. When we finally understand the fatal prehistory of the plot (hinted at through the flashbacks to Francis's joyful wife and daughter in a photograph and in the video scene, and to the search in a sunny field), we realise that at its core lies Francis's experience of being betrayed by his wife, through her affair with his brother Harold (Victor Garber). The subsequent deaths of their daughter Lisa, and of the wife herself, lead Francis to exploit both Christina and his niece Tracey (Sara Poley) in his attempt to recreate the yearned-for past. Harold—out of guilt—appears to sacrifice his daughter Tracey, allowing her to go to Francis for make-believe babysitting (a variation on the Dora theme). When Eric (Elias Koteas) jealously attempts to free Christina of her bond with Francis, he deceives Francis by luring him to touch Christina, so he can brutally throw him out of the club. In his attempted revenge, Francis blackmails Thomas—threatening to expose his illegal operations—into extracting the truth from Christina, and then wants to blackmail Thomas to help him murder Eric.

The manipulation of the other is more than exploitation here: the protagonists recreate each other, each becoming a construct in the other's inner reality. In the airport scene, Thomas closely observes his own image in the mirror, but behind his reflection in that one-way mirror hides Ian (Calvin Green), who is drawn to him. As the plot thickens, Christina becomes Lisa, the murdered girl (when performing, she wears a tartan skirt and a white blouse like Lisa, the film's ghostly apparition—Borden, 2000); Tracey takes the place of ex-babysitter Christina; Eric becomes the new murderer of the daughter (by destroying the bond between Francis and Christina); Thomas turns into Eric by finding the murdered daughter once more (as Eric found Lisa). The relationships between the figures are transferential, often projective, creating a complex chain of fantasy strings that eventually are all tied together masterfully.

But once more, on a deeper level, this world of fluid inter-changeable identities, of deception and manipulation, ultimately ends up being radically reversed, allowing 'something that feels vaguely like redemption' (Pevere, 1995, p. 36).

A crucial transformation takes place towards the end of the film. Francis's threat of turning Thomas in as a tax-evader was enough to send Thomas to tape Christina secretly and expose Eric; but when Francis wants his help to kill Eric, Thomas refuses. 'Not even to save a few years in prison?' Francis asks. 'No!' Thomas answers. 'Well, to help me then?'

Once we understand that Thomas agreed because he was moved by Francis's agony, a cynical view of human reality as based on power, exploitation and cold interests is no longer tenable. Help, caring, friendship turn out—after all—to be a real possibility. The agreement between Tracey and Francis to stop the pseudo-babysit-ting, and Christina's tears when Thomas wants to talk with her, also indicate that sincere expression makes a difference, that a talk-ing cure is possible.

Exotica follows an opposite path to that of the conventional detective film. Instead of moving from seeming innocence towards a discovery of guilt, it moves from a dark cloud of guilt (epitomised in the police's suspicion that Francis murdered Lisa, because he thought she was his brother's child) towards a discovery of total innocence. The film exonerates Francis more fully than the police ever could, because it allows him a chance to be eventually liberated from his inner guilt and self-doubt.

This reversal reaches its moving peak in the embrace between Eric and Francis. When Francis realises it was Eric who had discovered the body of his murdered daughter, he also understands that Eric has known and understood everything about him all along. Now, the manipulations both of them have used become trivial. They see each other, discover the deep bond uniting them: their partnership in the same tragedy, which has changed the lives of both. Instead of killing Eric, Francis finds himself hugging him. Treason and rage are transformed into compassion and mercy.

This breakthrough forces us to reconsider what we initially experienced as the perverse content of the film. We understand now that *Exotica* is at its core a film about unbearable catastrophic trauma, and about the convoluted but creative ways people find to deal with trauma, in order not to be petrified having watched Medusa's head. It is about the heavy baggage people carry, and about trying not to let it annihilate relationships and life, as Francis explains to Tracey when she brings up the tension between him and her father. 'How can people touch each other?' the film asks; 'What do they have to undergo in order to touch each other?' In spite of its story, and in spite of the nudity, *Exotica* is overall not a sexually stimulating film, but it ends up being emotionally stimulating in an unforeseen way.

We come to realise that neo-sexuality (McDougall, 1986) here is a way of handling traumatic baggage: inventing oneself anew in a way that will allow emotion and passion to survive in hiding, in spite of unbearable pain. Francis and Christina invent their ritual for that purpose. Now Francis is the omnipotent rescuer, which he failed to be for his actual daughter. Christina—who witnessed the discovery of Lisa's body, though Eric embraced her and so stopped her from watching the horror directly—invents herself as the innocent/sexy schoolgirl for Francis's sake. She is trying to cure him, and the club owner Zoe (Arsinée Khanjian) is alarmed: 'We are here to entertain, not to heal'.

What appeared as perverse sexual exploitation was actually a mutually constructed therapeutic mission. Eric diabolically destroyed this therapy by enticing Francis into a forbidden touch, a 'boundary violation'; but irrespective of his conscious motive, he was actually helping Francis and Christina to transcend a relationship that became ritualistically ossified. ('The problem with creating your own therapeutic exercises is that there's not someone there to monitor it ... to tell you if it's going too far ... Eric actually becomes a monitor for Francis', Egoyan, 1995, p. 55).

Egoyan's fascination with psychotherapy ('if I wasn't making films, maybe I'd be a therapist, because it's incredible to me that people go and spend an hour every week or day trying to work out something'; Egoyan, 1995, p. 55) goes hand in hand with sharp intuitive insights. Discussing his inspiration for *Exotica*, he says: 'During my adolescence I was very involved with somebody whom I later found out was being abused while I was involved with her ... There was a tremendous loneliness in the process of sexual communion ... That confusion has left a very deep impression on me ... somebody who is abused makes a parody of their own sexual identity as a means of trying to convince themselves that that part of themselves that has been destroyed is somehow not as vital as it is ... otherwise it becomes too painful' (1995, p. 48).

How reminiscent this is of Ferenczi's thinking about the aftermath of traumatic abuse (e.g. '*Posttraumatic effect*: identifications ... instead of one's own life', 1932, p. 171). The ritual was needed by

Christina too: 'I need him for certain things, and he needs me for certain things'. Egoyan sees the artificiality involved; his protagonists direct their own films. But he does not judge their imaginative dramatisation. In fact, he is also intrigued by its ultimate force: 'there's something fascinating about the fact that we do engineer sexual situations that we do lose ourselves in. Like a fetishist or sadomasochist or transvestite does—these are people I'm in awe of' (1995, p. 54).

Here, as elsewhere, Egoyan casts doubt upon any conventional boundary between normal and abnormal, between the despicable and the admirable.

In pointing, in its final scene, towards an earlier period in which Francis had been a benign father-figure for Christina, before his world collapsed, the film adds depth to its exploration of the role of sexuality in parental feelings. The intimacy between Francis and teenage Christina, when he drives her home after babysitting, has erotic undertones, but also a warm, caring, non-exploitative quality. Francis speaks admiringly of Lisa; Christina is moved. He says he is sure her parents talk about her that way too. 'I don't think so', she answers laconically. Francis mentions that Lisa says Christina really listens to her, but thinks she is not very happy. Christina appears to be on the verge of tears. He encourages her to talk to him about what might be going on at home. She doesn't, but says she enjoys the rides with him. She sadly goes out of his car, and walks slowly towards a big suburban house, into which she disappears.

This is an ominous, scary scene, more than any other part of *Exotica*. The film's protagonists are often eccentrics and outsiders (Zoe and Thomas appear to be immigrants in Canada, Francis's wife was black, Lisa mulatto—facts that are never mentioned, but play a role).[2] Nevertheless, their exotic 'otherness' is by now deconstructed; we understand them, we can empathise with their complex humanity. Christina's unseen (and unseeing?) parents now appear as the potential source of evil.

The real exotic horror does not reside in seedy nightclubs; it resides in the apparent respectability of the impenetrable suburban family home.

REFERENCES

BORDEN, D. (2000). Ritual haunting and the return of the depressed in Egoyan's *Exotica*. Paper presented at the Susan Zuckerman Memorial Program on Psychoanalysis and Cinema, San Francisco.

CURRENT BIOGRAPHY (1994). *Atom Egoyan*, 55: 155–60.

DONOVAN, W. (2000). *Exotica*: The privileges of otherness. Paper presented at the Susan Zuckerman Memorial Program on Psychoanalysis and Cinema, San Francisco.

---

[2] Egoyan's Armenian immigrant background, and his complex attitude towards it (forgetting the Armenian language as a child, intense reconnection from college on), are central in his life and work (*Current Biography*, 1994; Pevere, 1995). Donovan (2000) discusses the outsider's point of view in *Exotica* (which was made in Canada in 1994) and the unique perspective it allows. Otherness and marginality here are not only ethnic but also sexual: fertility belongs to pregnant Zoe, who appears to be bisexual, and to the smuggled exotic eggs connecting two homosexuals, Thomas and Ian (Borden, 2000).

EGOYAN, A. (1995). *Exotica.* Toronto: Coach House Press.

FERENCZI, S. (1932). *Clinical Diary,* ed. J. Dupont. Cambridge, MA: Harvard Univ. Press, 1988.

MCDOUGALL, J. (1986). Identifications, neoneeds and neosexualities. *Int. J. Psychoanal.,* 67: 19–31.

PEVERE, G. (1995). No place like home: the films of Atom Egoyan. Introduction to *Exotica,* by A. Egoyan. Toronto: Coach House Press, pp. 9–41.

23. THE REAL THING? SOME THOUGHTS ON *BOYS DON'T CRY*

DONALD MOSS AND LYNNE ZEAVIN, NEW YORK

Boys Don't Cry, written and directed by Kimberley Pierce, is a film provoked by the 1993 rape and murder of Teena Brandon/Brandon Teena, a 21-year-old transsexual. Brandon was killed in rural Nebraska, to which he had fled from Lincoln, where, Pierce sketchily, and light-heartedly, informs us, life had been laced with the intermittent pleasures and steady difficulties of trying to live as though a boy. Once relocated, Brandon won the friendship of a number of the town's young men, and the love of one of its most desired young women. When Brandon's neurotic penchant for acting out leads to yet another brief stay in a local jail, personal history and biological gender combine to expose her. This exposure eventually leads to her rape and murder.

Pierce, a New Yorker, dropped everything to attend the trial and, for months afterwards, lived amongst people who had constituted Brandon's last circle of intimates. The film, then, is a kind of case report. But rather than primarily study Brandon's transsexuality, the film presents her transsexual inclinations as a series of euphoric conquests. The film focuses on a range of anxious reactions to her transsexuality. Its strategy is comparable, perhaps, to using the particulars of the Dora case not for what they might reveal about female hysteria, but for what they might reveal about misogyny. The internal anguish wrought by and determining Brandon's sexual confusion is mostly left for the viewer to imagine and fill in. This gap will be particularly noticeable to a clinically inclined viewer. As viewers, we are given only intermittent glimpses into the costs of Brandon's daily sexual transgressions. These glimpses are, in part, meant to remind us of the costs of our own daily economies of transgression and compliance.

In her film, Pierce inserts the unconventional problems of transsexuality into a conventional narrative structure. Throughout the film Brandon is presented as a doomed, though beguiling and beautiful rascal, recognisably located in the lineage of well-known cinematic bad-boys like James Dean, Steve McQueen and Paul Newman. Like these predecessors, Brandon's heroic stature derives from her unwillingness to compromise her identity. Unlike them, though, the identity in question is in an unremitting and overt 'sexual crisis'. Pierce presents Brandon's struggles against biological determinism as the struggles of a dignified renegade.

Brandon's exhilarated state breaks down rarely in the film. The most poignant moments come when she is about to be revealed as a girl, or, more precisely, as a person with female genitals. Her euphoria is protected only while she can hide, and jeopardised only when her genitals might be seen by attacking men, by an examining doctor, or by her lover. These encounters between two different kinds of reality—one insistent upon hiding and one upon exposure—bring home the enormity of Brandon's crisis. The film presents these crises as taking place in a transitional zone. Rather than focus on the problems of Brandon's isolated, private, and tortured, sexual identity, Pierce highlights the culture-wide problems associated with separating sexual identity from genital anatomy.

The weight of Brandon's masquerade does not break her. We see her manage it strategically—tampons stolen from a drug store and carefully placed out of sight, her body 'strapped and packed' for every encounter. From the standpoint of the film, what demands accounting for is not her 'masquerade', but rather the indignation and, finally, the murderous rage that the masquerade provokes.

In the most thoroughgoing psychoanalytic encounters, as our patients recount their more or less effective efforts to mitigate what Freud called 'the bitter experience of life', we painfully bear witness to the eventual capitulation of fantasies to what seems like material necessity. We bear similar witness when watching Pierce's film. Pierce presents Brandon as the incarnation of the elementally Utopian, and classically tragic, hope in the triumph of psychic over material reality. Bearing such helpless witness, whether as clinicians or citizens, compels us to think of our own complicity in the usually latent violence by which cultural order is maintained and its renegades punished.

Once Brandon makes it out of Lincoln, the film focuses on his relationships with five people there—two male friends, a female lover, the lover's mother and a female friend. When Brandon, whom the five have all warmly received as a boy, is discovered to have a female body, each of the relationships is put into crisis. The varying responses seem intended to mark out a full range of possibilities. The female friend feels betrayed but remains sympathetic, perhaps pitying. The female lover remains adamant; no matter the genital particulars—for her, Brandon was, is, and will always be a boy. The mother is disgusted; the figure she once adored as so 'handsome' is now transformed into someone 'sick' and despicable; she is indifferent to his fate. The two male friends feel they have been lied to, deceived; they react vengefully, furiously, first with rape, and then, when Brandon informs the police, with murder. These are the reactions that the audience must work to comprehend. Something about Brandon's comfort with her own erotic fluidity unearths the violence in these men. Anything but erotically fluid themselves, they each seem, instead, to be stuck in extremely restrictive prototypical versions of masculinity. For both, erotic competence is lived out, lock-step, primarily in the form of a preening, aggressive meanness—a competence grounded in resentful submission to the way things have to be. Meanness and resentment provide contact points for mutual identification and an effective cover for mutual love. Men are the primary audience for other men's preening. They alone are endowed with the power to judge each other's claim to be 'real' men. The film vividly illuminates this in a rodeo scene where men ride the tailgates of careening pick-up trucks so as to demonstrate their heterosexual virility to other men. The scene conveys a circus atmosphere—masculine exhibition, and an excited male audience. Women, meanwhile, occupy the position of mere coin in this barely concealed homoerotic economy. Brandon's erotic deftness, her capacities to 'pass' the rodeo test and still remain tuned in to feminine desire, exposes both the restrictive and the homoerotic dimensions of the oppressive masculinity with which these men are saddled. They want to pay her back and do it on sexual terms. Together, each the other's witness, they rape her, in an act of violence that seems intended to simultaneously affirm and deny their erotic commitments to each other while teaching Brandon and her friends a female's proper place, when Brandon, by pressing charges, resists the lesson, they kill her.

Pierce uses these five relationships to interrogate the structural interrelations linking identity to normativity, power to desire, sexual fantasy to genital endowment, and truth to violence. The film is organised around the reactions to the discovery of Brandon's genital status. As such, the particular focus of the film's enormously dense agenda is on the contested relation between sexual authenticity and sexual masquerade. Pierce directs us, as viewers, away from the usual subject–object position underlying film spectatorship. We identify with Brandon, and with this, that traditional relation has been transformed into an identification. Dislodged from our customary position, we thus feel ourselves participating in the belief/delusion of Brandon's status as a boy. When we watch Brandon undress we find ourselves believing, with her, that in spite of anatomy, we are seeing the body of a boy. And when anatomy makes its claims on our eyes we wonder, with Brandon, how best to resist them. This internal conflict between perception and idea, in turn, reveals much about our assumptions concerning gender and gender prerogatives. Such is the driving effort of Pierce's film—to expose our desires and our hatreds even while it protects Brandon's from more exacting scrutiny.

Brandon's life history, as presented by Pierce, leads us to again assess the shifting balance of forces underlying the relations between sexual identity and genital anatomy, psychic reality and material reality. For Pierce, none of the elements constituting those relations are fixed. This is made clear by her intense focus on the ongoing interpersonal elements that dog each transsexually laden encounter.

The film's material, then, both derives from and illuminates features of the contemporary debates on sexuality that are enlivening both contemporary psychoanalysis and the culture at large. The ever-widening scope of this contemporary debate, instigated within psychoanalysis first by feminist and then by gay and lesbian activists, centres on the reading of the relations between sexual 'difference' and sexual deviance. The debate as presented by Pierce coincides with and illuminates the two apparently irreconcilable promises of an ongoing debate within psychoanalysis.

One premise reads the periphery—difference and deviance—from the vantage-point of a posited centre. That posited centre gives this reading its elemental point of stability and coherence. In principle, from this point of view, difference, as such, is distance from the centre, and distance, when marked, is deviance. From here, the centre is not the product of circumstance or convention; rather, it is the product of law, of necessity. Within psychoanalysis, a most articulate spokesperson of this point of view is Janine Chasseguet-Smirgel.

The other premise reads the centre from the point of view of the periphery. The centre, then, becomes merely a 'centre', a construction. From here, the pertinent task is not, primarily, a critical assessment of deviance, but rather a critical assessment of the centre's claims—its metaphysical sense of itself, and of the norms grounded in this metaphysics—phallocentrism, logocentrism, Eurocentrism etc. From the periphery, the centre ought not to serve as theory's source, but rather as theory's object. Difference, in principle, is to be read as a marker of multiplicity rather than of deviance. Here, we might locate the representative voices of Thomas Ogden, say, and Jessica Benjamin.

This contemporary debate, with all of its baroque postmodern turns, is a continuation of the one from which Freud extracted the elementary tenets of clinical psychoanalysis a century ago. It is one measure of the merit of *Boys Don't Cry* that both the problems it addresses and the rhetorical and narrative strategies it employs bear comparison to the problems faced and the strategies he used in writing his foundational text, *Three Essays on the Theory of Sexuality* (1905, *S.E.* 7).

Freud's *Three Essays* ... are a marvel of rhetorical cunning. They invite the reader to participate in what seems a traditional and conservative approach to the so-called 'sexual deviations'. But Freud finally, and subtly, turns the entire classificatory project around on itself. Essays that begin by accepting the established divide between the classifying subject and the deviant object end by asserting a covert relation binding deviation to normality. While the traditional strategy of classification leads to a localisation and externalisation of deviance, Freud's leads to a universalisation and internalisation of it. If the deviant is enacting what the classifiers fantasise, then the direct classification of manifest sexual deviance will correspond to an indirect classification of neurotic fantasy. Freud's essays have the effect of moving his reader from the secure position of disinterested subject to the less secure one of implicated object.

Like Freud's *Three Essays*, *Boys Don't Cry* is a rhetorically sophisticated look at sexual deviance. The film's sophistication, like Freud's, is grounded in its reversal of normative grounding premises. Traditionally, transsexuals are situated as 'cases', people whose problematic sexuality potentially assists us in our ongoing effort at mapping the relations between sexuality and gender, mind and body, fantasy and reality. Like Freud, Pierce inverts the framing question. Freud established sexuality as the independent, and universal, variable and charted its formal variations in subjects and objects. Pierce presents transsexuality as a kind of unloosed sexuality, a sexuality apparently shorn of material constraint, and of all the signifiers that usually clothe it in reasonableness. She then charts the formal variations this wild card provokes in affected subjects and objects.

As did Freud, Pierce directs our attention not to an interrogation of the unbound sexual constant, but rather of its bound, and inconstant, variations. She wants us to ask: given the disruptions of an unadorned, tyrannical sexuality, what are the determinants that provoke disgust here, hatred there, violence there, love here; an affirmation of psychic over material reality here, its reverse there? As did Freud, Pierce uses such questions to illuminate the faultlines that undermine our every sense of sexual certainty. After all, Pierce seems to suggest, leaning this time on both Flaubert and Freud, for all of us, to the extent that we are all sexual, '*Teena Brandon/Brandon Teena, c'est nous*'.

24. FIFTEEN MINUTES OF FAME REVISITED: *BEING JOHN MALKOVICH*

GLEN O. GABBARD, Topeka, KS

In the closing lines of Philip Roth's *The Counterlife* (1986), Nathan Zuckerman reluctantly concludes, 'It may be as you say that this is no life, but use your enchanting, enrapturing brains: This life is as close to life as you, and I, and our child could ever hope to come' (p. 324). This sobering resignation to life-as-it-is comes at the end of a novel in which the characters have relentlessly searched for an alternative existence that might reverse their fate. The theme of throwing off the shackles of one's apparently meaningless life and undergoing a miraculous transformation into another person is a ubiquitous motif in literature and film. Indeed, our understanding of the psychoanalytic concept of projective identification owes a debt to the Julian Green novella, *If I Were You*, in which the protagonist vacates his own body to inhabit the minds of others. Klein's classic 1955 paper, 'On identification', places this novella at the centre of her exposition.

A recent cinematic variation on this theme was the 1999 winner of the National Society of Film Critics' Best Picture Award, *Being John Malkovich*. Directed by Spike Jonze and written by Charlie Kaufman, the film tells the story of a beleaguered puppeteer named Craig Schwartz (John Cusack). He likes puppeteering, he says, because it enables him to place himself in someone else's skin for a while. Stuck in a dreary marriage to his drab and animal-obsessed wife Lotte (Cameron Diaz), Craig lives a life of quiet desperation. In the opening minutes of the film he says, 'Consciousness is a terrible curse. I think, I feel, I suffer'.

Craig's transcendence of his despair begins when he applies for a filing job in a New York office building. To his dismay he discovers that there is no elevator button for the seventh-and-a-half floor where the office is housed. A good Samaritan riding with him in the elevator turns on the alarm button to stop the elevator between the seventh and eighth floors. Craig emerges into this space between floors, and he soon discovers that it is also a transitional space between illusion and reality. The ceilings are so low that he has to walk in an uncomfortable bent-over position. The receptionist in the office cannot hear, and her boss (Orson Bean) assumes that he must have a speech impediment because she cannot understand him.

In this transitional arena the film takes a Lewis Carroll turn when Craig, like the heroine of *Alice in Wonderland*, discovers a portal in the wall that leads to an alternative reality. At the other end of the portal is an entry into the head of the actor John Malkovich. The inhabitation of the actor lasts only fifteen minutes, after which Craig is deposited alongside the New Jersey Turnpike.

Ecstatic about his new-found potential for self-transcendence, Craig enlists the help of his office colleague Maxine (Catherine Keener) to exploit the portal for fun and profit. They call their company 'JM Inc.', and the marketing slogan is 'Have you ever wanted to be someone else?' Soon the denizens of New York City are lining up for an opportunity to spend fifteen minutes as John Malkovich.

This fulfilment of Andy Warhol's prediction that in the future everyone will become famous for fifteen minutes becomes a marvellous satire on the emptiness of celebrity. Through ingenious use of the camera, Jonze allows us to see what the world looks like through the eyes of a famous person. The visual portrait is stunning in its ordinariness. The world looks exactly like it does when we look through our own eyes. As Chang notes in his analysis of the film, 'The bottom line, in the film's version of reality, is that Malkovich is neither more nor less than any of the anonymous humans who pass through life without the benefit of limelit incandescence. We are just too blinded by the stars to realize it' (1999, p. 9). At the climax of the film when Malkovich (played by himself) discovers what is going on, he enters the portal himself, only to discover that through Malkovich's eyes, everyone looks exactly like Malkovich, talks exactly like Malkovich, and has the content of their speech limited to the word 'Malkovich'.

This hilarious parody of celebrity narcissism raises a myriad of questions about why Malkovich was selected and why he agreed to join the project. A running gag throughout the film involves the fact that no one really knows who he is. In fact, he is the ultimate inkblot. A cab driver refers to him as 'John Mapplethorpe' and thinks he was in a jewel thief film (which he was not). When Craig shares his discovery with Maxine, her response is, 'Who the fuck is John Malkovich?'

While Jonze and Kaufman have been fairly inscrutable in interviews, the actor has been much more forthcoming. John Malkovich himself embodies a sense of self-parody. When asked if he approached the role differently from the way he would another character, he wryly responded, 'Without being too polemical, I don't really think of myself as John Malkovich' (Lim, 1999). In his own way, the actor communicates that his sense of who he is bears almost no relation to the celebrity version of John Malkovich. The screenplay supports him in this regard, as the character Malkovich is seen as nothing more than another puppet, a vessel that others inhabit, a container imbued with the idealising transference of ordinary non-celebrities. At one point Maxine asks Craig, 'Is he appealing?' Craig responds, 'Of course, he's a celebrity'.

Kaufman suggests that the character Malkovich is not the real Malkovich through subtle changes in biographical details. Although the film portrays Malkovich as having been born in Evanston, Illinois, and attending Northwestern University, neither of those biographical details is actually true. Nor does the emptiness of the character Malkovich match the archness and slightly reprehensible seediness that we have come to associate with the actor Malkovich (at least as we think we know him). Recognition of the difference between actor and character was perhaps best embodied in the fact that the New York film critics gave Malkovich the Best Supporting Actor award—the first and probably only time that an actor will be awarded for playing himself.

The actor John Malkovich, always sceptical of celebrity, appears to be deeply committed to the message of the film: 'I think there's a need for us to escape ourselves for some period of time, escape our existence, our ridiculousness, our nature. And there's the idea that a celebrity's blowjobs are interesting and yours aren't, which our culture insists on as a constitutional right and our media promulgates in the most vicious, irresponsible, ludicrous, cynical way' (Lim, 1999).

While the audience can clearly see that there is nothing particularly spectacular about being in John Malkovich's head, the characters are blind to the fact that his existence varies little from their own. Craig's wife Lotte exclaims, 'Being inside did something to me. I knew who I was'. She sexualises the experience, referring to the portal as 'like a vagina', and decides that she must be a transsexual because it felt so right to be in a man's body. She then engages in an intense sexual relationship with Maxine, but only when she is in Malkovich's body. Screenwriter Kaufman then has a good deal of fun spoofing the postmodern sensibility of multiple selves and gender-bending. Jonze even throws in an amusing jab at psychoanalysis when Lotte and Maxine go through the portal together and enter the unconscious of Malkovich, where he is a little boy standing in his parents' bedroom and observing the primal scene.

As the film winds towards its ending, a group of elderly body-snatchers await immortality by jumping from body to body. Craig begins to realise that switching bodies may not be the answer to all of one's problems and appears to reach a conclusion that closely resembles Zuckerman's sobering realisation in *The Counterlife*— that although we would like to leave ourselves behind, we are more or less stuck with the life that we have been given and might as well enjoy it. The irony of this message is that it is delivered to a group of people in a darkened cinema who are there for the same reason that characters in the film line up at the portal. They wish to be transported out of themselves into a celluloid world that only bears a marginal relation to reality. Martin Scorsese's *King of Comedy* (1983) and several films in Woody Allen's canon, including *Stardust Memories* (1980), *Zelig* (1983), *The Purple Rose of Cairo* (1985) and *Celebrity* (1998), have made similar points about the shallowness of celebrity (Gabbard & Gabbard, 1999). Yet audiences don't necessarily listen to the message these films convey. Somehow we cannot entirely accept that the life we have is as good as it gets, and the need to transcend ourselves and to believe in the illusion that others are different from us may be central to some form of redemption in our secular age. In the absence of a portal, we line up at the box office.

REFERENCES

CHANG, C. (1999). Head wide open. *Film Comment*, 35: 6–9.

GABBARD, G. O. & GABBARD, K. (1999). *Psychiatry and the Cinema.* Washington, DC: American Psychiatric Press, 2nd edn.

KLEIN, M. (1955). On identification. In *Envy and Gratitude and Other Works, 1946–1963*. New York: Delacorte Press/Seymour Laurence, 1975, pp. 141–75.

LIM, D. (1999). Brain humor. *The Village Voice*, October 20–26 http://www.villagevoice.com/issues/9942/lim.shtml

ROTH, P. (1986). *The Counterlife*. New York: Farrar, Straus & Giroux.

25. *THE SIXTH SENSE*

PHILIP A. RINGSTROM, Encino, CA

M. Night Shyamalan's *The Sixth Sense* (1999) is about the terrifying consequences of being unwilling to look at critically important truths about oneself. The film also explores the transformative experience that ensues when one finally looks at those truths and actually grasps them. The methodological schema employed in this review is 'the analysis of spectatorship'—that is, 'the engagement of the audience member's perspective, as if the camera itself' (Gabbard, 1997, p. 4). Though the element of spectatorship pervades the film, it achieves its most powerful and undeniable moment in the final scene, which therefore requires exposition at the beginning of this essay to establish a context of interpretation for the film as a whole.

In the film's final moments, a shocking revelation simultaneously assaults Dr Malcolm Crow (Bruce Willis), and the audience. Dr Crow is dead. He turns out to be one of many traumatised ghosts who wander in torment until the source of what haunts them is discovered. Particularly bedevilling to these lost souls is the fact that they do not know they are ghosts. Dr Crow's 9-year-old patient Cole (Haley Joel Osment) explains to his divorced, single-parent mother (Toni Collette), 'They only see what they want to see'. The spectral twist in the narrative of the film is that Cole's observation is no less applicable to those of us who are watching the film. We too are ultimately shocked by Dr Crow's death because we too see only what we want to see!

Shyamalan, who does double duty as screenwriter and director, is a master illusionist. He understands that if you supply even the slightest detail of a desired version of reality, your audience will supply the rest. Wishes dictate what is seen; denial keeps the undesired at bay. Shyamalan keenly grasps that the latter corresponds with our collective denial of death, while the former reflects our wish for resurrection, or more simply put, to get a second chance.

In the first scene, we are immediately lured into Shyamalan's web of illusions. Dr Malcolm Crow and his wife Anna are at home celebrating his Mayor's citation for professional excellence from the city of Philadelphia for his personal sacrifices as a child psychologist. Their inebriated celebration is punctuated by a former child patient—now young adult—named Vincent Grey (Donnie Wahlberg) breaking into their upstairs bedroom. In a horrific confrontation, Vincent first lambasts Dr Crow for his failure to help him as a child and then shoots Crow in the abdomen. Crow's former patient caps this violent act by putting a bullet through his own head.

The scene that immediately follows is captioned, 'The Next Fall; South Philadelphia'. Dr Crow, apparently alive and well, is sitting outside a city block of row houses reading handwritten case notes regarding what we presume to be his next child patient, 9-year-old Cole. This moment fulfils the audience's fervent wish for Crow to get his 'second chance'.

The viewers of this film are similarly 'taken in' a short while later at an initial psychotherapy session involving a home visit. Cole's mother and Dr Crow are sitting face to face in her living room as Cole returns home from school. The surprising revelation to many who saw the film a second time is that Dr Crow and Cole's mother are silent throughout the scene. Cole's mother clearly has no awareness of Dr Crow. Indeed, her look is one of an anxious mother awaiting her ill son's safe arrival home. Shyamalan further dupes the audience with the mother's bit of playful bantering in which she says, 'You've got an hour' (before supper), appearing to knowingly leave Cole and Dr Crow to their first encounter. Her throwaway comment supplies coherence to what we want to believe, that she was alluding to a therapy hour.

Cole is tormented by the fact that he is able to see things that others cannot bear to see. This 'sixth sense' is his gift, or perhaps his curse. As the camera allows the audience to witness the macabre ghosts he sees, we become engrossed in the terrifying consequences for both the ghosts and ultimately for young Cole. In the absence of the knowledge that they are dead, they are compelled to walk the earth in a painful form of dissociated self-deception. Their agonising effect upon Cole derives from his own failed attempts to engage in a similar form of self-deception. As audience members, we are unwittingly on the verge of grasping an important truth; namely, that when deception prevents us from seeing the truth about ourselves, about others, or about both, trauma likely ensues. Indeed, we learn from each new encounter with a ghost that it was their neglect of this truth that brought on their own traumatic deaths, and their unwillingness to recognise this neglect haunts them in perpetuity.

Wise beyond his years, Cole understands this but is helpless to do anything about it. He too is traumatised during every waking moment, knowing he may encounter yet another anguished ghost. When Dr Crow arrives as his would-be psychological healer, an initially suspicious Cole begins to intuitively grasp that this ghost might be able to help him, but only if he too can find a way to heal his healer. Cole's challenge is to heal Crow while illuminating a critical truth about himself that he does not grasp.

Cole realises that since ghosts do not want to know who and what they are, he must gently unveil this fact to Dr Crow. First Cole must convince the doubting Dr Crow that he (Cole) actually does see ghosts. An important, but perhaps unintended, message here is that no therapist can help his patient unless he can find something plausible in his patient's story. Only when Crow embraces the boy's story is he able to convince Cole that he must no longer flee into his protective bedspread-erected sanctuary, but instead must face the ghosts. We, like Crow, however, do not yet know the ultimate truth. We wish for his redemption and for the salvation of Cole. We eagerly embrace his intervention when Dr Crow tells Cole, 'I think I know how to help them (the ghosts) go away ... just listen to them'.

To our collective relief, Dr Crow's admonition works. Finally, Cole is able to listen to a teenage ghost named Kira, and Cole helps her expose how her Munchausen-deranged mother slowly and accidentally poisoned her to death in an attempt to forestall Kira's separation and individuation. His action brings peace to the tormented teenage ghost while saving Kira's younger sister from what appears to be an inevitably similar fate.

Cole's liberation now readies him to become his therapist's therapist. We begin to discover that 9-year-old Cole has an intuitive grasp of good analytic technique. Cole never directly tells his 'patient' Dr Crow, 'You are a ghost'. Instead, he deftly enables Crow to arrive at his own ineluctable conclusion.

Returning to the final scene, when Dr Crow recovers from what is his own, not to mention the audience's, shocking discovery that he is dead, he applies the cryptic intervention his young mentor taught him. He speaks to Anna in her sleep and tells her something he had not yet been able to articulate, namely, that she was never 'second' in importance to him. Like the ghosts in Thorton Wilder's *Our Town*, his universal message speaks to all of us who have placed the person we most love second in our attention. By his revelation, Dr Crow is finally set free, and so too is Anna.

The film's message is both timeless and simple: the truth will set you free. It brilliantly underscores that people at risk of embodying living deaths prefer to believe that which they want to, rather than what they need to be set free. The final most haunting question is more complex: set free to do what? Shyamalan understands that this conundrum, when addressed head-on, is too easily dismissed. One dimension of his genius is how he makes an unbearable but ineluctable truth creep into us without our noticing. Though his message may have originated outside of us, by drawing us in as spectators who are literally in the dark, his film's haunting truth becomes inescapable. The ghost of trauma perpetually torments us in our denial, until we awaken to our problems.

REFERENCE

GABBARD, G. (1997). The psychoanalyst at the movies. *Int. J. Psychoanal.*, 78: 1–6.